Advance Praise

Client endorsers have been assured confidentiality

"I have struggled with infertility for 3 years and have had a history of recurrent losses. I am still on my journey. Along the way, I have become discouraged, hopeless, and even depressed. I started to realize that my emotions and attitudes were getting in the way of my living life, and I somehow stumbled upon Rosanne Austin's Fearlessly Fertile Method. I only wish I found Rosanne Austin sooner. She has really helped to normalize some of my emotions and reframe my thoughts. As a physician and patient, I know that medicine doesn't solve everything and there are still a lot of factors out there that we can't explain. I feel healthier and more positive by using her strategies. I feel less anxious and jealous. I feel I have personally grown through her advice. She is real and honest. This book is a quick read, but packs a lot of punch. It provides a great foundation for anyone struggling with the emotional aspect of infertility."

–Dr. Michelle Y.

"Highly recommend this book for anyone struggling on their fertility journey. I was so excited when I heard Rosanne was coming out with a book. She is the real deal and when you follow her teachings that she shares in her book you will find success. I was very lucky to have worked with Rosanne on my own journey of becoming a mom I am not only pregnant for the very first time after years of TTC (now 26 weeks pregnant), but she taught me a new way to live. In this book you will find all the tools that you will need to turn around your fertility nightmare into your fertility dream. Just like us, Rosanne knows the fertility struggle, she can relate with us and in this book she uses a sense of humor and teaching style that is inspiring and not overwhelming. Best of luck on your fertility journey and I hope you fall in love with this book as much as I have."

–Jennifer Z.

"Rosanne's book is amazing. Based on her own experience, she wrote a playbook that empowered me to see things clearly for the very first time though I thought I knew it all. Her ideas plus the helpful exercises changed the outlook on my fertility journey. In only a couple of days, communication between my husband and I improved. We're much closer now; I have become really optimistic and discovered that I am not helpless. I feel more at ease than ever and started to rejoice that my baby is coming. The Fearlessly Fertile Method is designed by a woman who is passionate about mindset and motherhood. She speaks from her heart in every word of this book. It will make you laugh a bit, cry a bit, and in the end you win."

–Hannah A.

"I discovered Rosanne Austin at the "perfect" time in my fertility journey. I was crushed with the fact that I could get pregnant, but couldn't stay pregnant. My only tool was my doctor, and I struggled with dismal statistics that were meant to encourage me. Rosanne's book created a-ha moments I know I need to make my motherhood dreams a reality. Ways to acknowledge statistics and keep moving toward my reality, encouragement to surround myself with the right people and ways to remember who I am as I jump through the hoops. I know my mindset is the key to holding my baby and I'm grateful to hold (and use) Rosanne's toolbox as I get closer to realizing my dream."

–Amy S.

"This is an amazing book written by a true godsend of a fertility mindset master, Rosanne Austin. I struggled to get pregnant for three years and had two failed IVFs. After practicing the exercises in this book, religiously, and following where they led me in my life, I became pregnant -NATURALLY. As Rosanne often says, this isn't hocus- pocus: it's the real deal. This book will show you how to remove the mental blocks that are standing in your way between you and your baby, and it'll make you believe you are meant to be a Mom (as Rosanne always says).

There are so many books out there that you can buy, but none of them have the passion, energy, and practical know-how that this one has. Rosanne just makes you feel so good about yourself and your ability to conceive, something we all feel starved of on this journey. And, she won't BS you by sugar coating things. The book asks you to do a lot of self-work, but the reward is immeasurable. I wish every woman struggling with fertility would pick this up and follow it. It changed my fertility journey and my life completely."

–Kathryn B.

"Saying that I felt Rosanne was in my head when she wrote this book would be a massive understatement. I'm also an alpha female that climbed the career ladder through hard work and dedication, married her soul-mate then expected babies to come as "planned"- only to experience the heartbreak and frustration of years of failed fertility treatments. And Rosanne GETS ME. The inspirational words and personal stories within these pages will undoubtedly create "aha" moments for any woman on her fertility journey. It also provides the tools to move forward with the heartfelt knowledge that motherhood IS ahead. As a woman that worked with Rosanne and implemented the Fearlessly Fertile Method in her life, I can tell you that not only will it help you rediscover the woman you know yourself to be, it can also lead you to your baby. It did for me - my little miracle arrived 1 month before my 41st birthday! Thank you, Rosanne, for pouring your heart and soul into these pages. My baby (who just turned 2) and her momma are eternally grateful!"

–Jessica S.

Am I The Reason I'm Not Getting Pregnant?

Am I the Reason I'm Not Getting Pregnant?

The **FEARLESSLY FERTILE™**
Method for Clearing the Blocks
Between You and Your Baby

ROSANNE AUSTIN

NEW YORK

LONDON • NASHVILLE • MELBOURNE • VANCOUVER

Am I the Reason I'm Not Getting Pregnant?

The Fearlessly Fertile™ Method for Clearing the Blocks Between You and Your Baby

Published in New York, New York, by Morgan James Publishing in partnership with Difference Press. Morgan James is a trademark of Morgan James, LLC. www.MorganJamesPublishing.com

ISBN 9781642798562 paperback
ISBN 9781642798579 eBook
ISBN 9781642798586 audiobook
Library of Congress Control Number: 2019951775

Cover & Interior Design by:
Christopher Kirk
www.GFSstudio.com

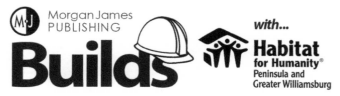

Morgan James is a proud partner of Habitat for Humanity Peninsula and Greater Williamsburg. Partners in building since 2006.

Get involved today! Visit
MorganJamesPublishing.com/giving-back

For Brandon and Asher, my living proof of miracles.

Table of Contents

Foreword

AM I THE REASON I'M NOT GETTING PREGNANT? *YES!* My comments about not getting pregnant aren't intended to create guilt or place blame, but to empower women. From my life's work I have seen the power of the mind and how it can repair and alter the body by the message it sends to the body. What you think and believe can have a profound effect on your body's ability to heal and function properly, which of course includes getting pregnant and carrying your baby to term. Beliefs can be powerful medicine.

Let me share some true stories that demonstrate this:

One of the nurses in our office confessed to me that she was having difficulties conceiving. She shared how her thoughts and feelings had become so negative. I told her to start visualizing herself becoming pregnant and to eliminate all the fears and negative images filling her mind. She started following my advice and within two weeks was pregnant.

I also remember working with a medical student to help him to decode what branch of medicine to specialize in. I asked him to draw pictures for me to illustrate what he wanted for his life. Several of his drawings showed a future family with three children. Years later after his graduation, we connected and he shared how his wife was having troubles conceiving. I found and showed him the drawings he had made of the family he had envisioned. I told him to focus on the vision he had for his family. I knew he and his wife would have the three children they envisioned one way or another, if they stayed committed to that vision. Several years later the news was that he and his wife had three children.

The most dramatic example of how powerful the mind can be in supporting pregnancy was the time I received a phone call from one of my patients telling me that she was in the hospital in premature labor. The doctors and everyone around her felt there was nothing more they could do to try and prevent a miscarriage. I went to her hospital room, which was so filled with despair and depression you could feel when you walked in. I blurted out to everyone, "Get out of here!" Their negativity was doing nothing for this woman. I scared the staff and family and they left. Then she and I did a meditation and imagery in which she visualized and communicated with her uterus, sending it love to get it to relax and stop contracting. Within fifteen minutes, her labor stopped and she went on to full term delivery. I later received a phone call from her to tell me they were naming the new baby boy after me, but since they were Irish his name was Brady—not Bernie.

I didn't just see the power of the mind have an impact on my patients' ability to have the babies they wanted I also saw it at work in my own family. My wife had incredible power over her mind and body. After having three boys, I asked her if we could get pregnant again, and try for a daughter. She agreed, knowing how much we wanted a daughter. Then came the surprise news was that she was carrying twins. I will never forget when she said, "If it's two more boys, I am not coming home from the hospital!" In those days we didn't have ultrasound, so there was no way of knowing the gender of the twins. When the babies were born, I heard the obstetrician say, "What a gentleman, he let his sister out first," I knew it was okay and that my lovely wife would be coming home!" We envisioned having a daughter and that is exactly what we did.

My wife also used the power of her mind to align the birth of our children with important dates in our lives. She had such control! I was born on the fourteenth and my wife on the ninth—so, I knew our first son would be born on the twenty-third. We were married on the eleventh, and our second son born on the twenty-second. Our third son was born on the third day of the eleventh month. The synchronicity was fascinating, but of course not surprising, knowing my wife. When my wife was pregnant with the twins, the delivery was near Christmas time and my wife said, "I will not be in the hospital on Christmas!" At that moment, I knew exactly when they were coming. Yup, December twenty-sixth.

By sharing these stories, it is my hope that you can see how influential you can be in your own healing. When you take control of your thoughts and beliefs, you can create peace of mind, which in turn creates a healing environment in the body. Anyone who is willing to work at it can achieve it. Having struggled with fertility herself, let what Rosanne teaches in this book inspire you and help you empower yourself to become the mother you were meant to be.

Bernie S. Siegel, MD

New York Times best-selling author of *Love, Medicine, and Miracles: Lessons Learned About Self-Healing from a Surgeon's Experience with Exceptional Patients*

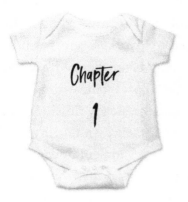

Chapter
1

Fertility Freak-Out Is Real ... *Real*

"It's better to look ahead and prepare
than to look back and regret."
— Jackie Joyner-Kersee

S omething tells me you never thought you'd find yourself reading a book like this – *about* this. As a little girl, you probably imagined that at this point in your life, you'd be riding high on decades of accomplishments, with the partner and house of your dreams, knowing that as long as you worked hard enough, you'd get what you want more likely than not. There's nothing quite like a struggle with fertility to call into question just about everything you believe about yourself as a woman, the control you have over your destiny, and the way the world is "supposed to" work. Even if you had a reason to suspect your fertility may be challenged, we tend to look at it as a *biological basic.* We expect that, with all the advances made in modern medicine and the steady flow of celebrities showing off baby bumps in spite of their own fertility challenges, we will be having a *Sound of Music* moment down diaper aisle at Target in no time after a minor tweak or two – until, of course, the tweaks we prepared for turn into repeated disappointments and failure.

I bet you've never felt like more of a failure in your life. And let's be honest, that's what it feels like. There's no use in sugarcoating it. Unlike everything you have done up to this point in your life, whether it was working on your education or climbing the ranks in your profession, you've never backed down from rolling up your sleeves and handling your business. In fact, you don't just get things done; you are at the top of your professional game. People know that when you are on the job, every *t* will be crossed and every *i* will be dotted. You are the go-to person when success is a nonnegotiable. You've earned a reputation for getting the job done right the first time. If only you felt that in control when it comes to your fertility!

As you've probably figured out by now, when it comes to your efforts to conceive, there is no direct correlation between how hard you "work" and the result you get. It's infuriating. In fact, it can seem like the harder you try, the more frustrating your results. You probably started out this journey gung-ho, ready to crush it, like you do everything else. Maybe you took the first few blows to the chin like a champ, shook them off, and chalked it up to timing or "bad luck." But as your disappointment and failures started piling up, the "I've got this" swagger that's served you so well in other aspects of your life darted out of the room and the stinking, icky desperation of "Why can't I catch a break?!" slithered right in. Powerlessness pushes every last one of your lovably type A, control-freaky, slightly obsessive, make-it-happen buttons. So, you spend hours replaying and reliving every possible misstep along the way, looking for any explanation for why even your best efforts are "failing." Determined to crack the fertility code, you double down on the discipline. You work even harder, try to be more perfect, and spend countless hours with your illicit lover Dr. Google, researching into the wee hours of the night until your eyes are practically bleeding, looking for *The Answer.* Such answers have proven to be elusive.

How Did This Become My Life?

Up to this point, you figured having a baby would be *part of* your life, not a pursuit that *became* your life. Even if you had some reason to believe your fertility could be an issue, never in your worst nightmares did you think you'd live in what feels like a permanent state of anxiety-laden chaos. Not only are you living your life in two-week increments, but it also feels like your entire life is structured around your next menstrual cycle or fertility treatment. The life you knew before this baby-making odyssey began seems like a distant, misty memory, along with the once carefree – "reckless" by comparison – lifestyle you used to lead. You long for the days of simple pleasures like gluten, dairy, sex just because it's awesome, and a healthy relationship with the sight of pregnant women.

What's crazy is that in many ways, it feels like you are living a double life. At work, your calm, cool, and collected exterior is a thin veneer over the deeply sensitive woman beneath whose heart is breaking with fear that she will never have the one thing she truly wants more than anything right now: her baby. The only real tip-off is you are missing more work than usual lately to make all of your doctor's appointments and other treatments. Only the nosiest of your coworkers would begin to put two and two together and speculate. They might start to suspect that you have some dreaded disease. In truth, as bitterly judgmental as it is, there's part of you that would rather they believed you were dying than ever find out you are failing at something "undeserving others" seem to do with ease.

As if things couldn't get more complicated, you find yourself trying to navigate the impact your fertility journey is having on the lives of the people closest to you – including your family and friends. Not wanting to burden anyone, you've been careful to keep the soul-searing pain of living virtually every day wondering if "it" will ever happen quietly tucked away. Your brave face is the stuff of legends. You endure their well-intentioned – but at times insensitive and grating – comments with decently good humor, but even that is wearing dangerously thin. You've gotten to the point where it's easier to just keep things to yourself than expend the energy trying to share this deeply emotional, intimate, and complex part of your life. It feels too vulnerable and raw. No matter how hard they try, they are not going to get it. Besides, crying in the shower is way more efficient and satisfying than having to explain this insanity to anyone.

With all of this going on, there's also the not-so-small matter of your partner. As loving, supportive, and awesome as your partner is, there are times when you catch them giving you a look like, "Is she crazy?" Since their fertility tests indicate no real issues, they seem to have the luxury of a decidedly more mellow take on things, which unintentionally adds to your stress. While things between you are still good, there's no denying the situation has changed. Sex feels contrived and there's an undeniable gray undercurrent of the unsaid. Trying to conceive has dominated the conversation for so long and has such a powerful grip on your lives that it's become easier to just repeat chipper platitudes or not say anything at all. Then of course there's the most unspeakable topic of all, "What if it doesn't work out for us?" Perhaps you've had a polite, hypothetical in nature, intellectual discussion of what your backup plan might be, but neither of you is particularly excited about going "there."

Feeling like there's pressure mounting on all sides, you go back to doing what you do best: trying harder, pushing farther, and doing "everything" you can. But nothing is working.

Doing Everything, *And Then Some*

In case anyone was wondering, the notion that you are doing "everything" is no exaggeration. From the moment your journey started it was *game on.* While you've always maintained a healthy lifestyle through diet and exercise, with your fertility at stake, you went full throttle, scorched earth, opting for the most agro, Puritanically clean diet you could get your hands on. For you, willpower is *not* an issue. You've got the stamina of a marathon runner, and there's no way on this green earth you're going to let something like an errant dietary choice stand between you and your rightful spot in the Mama-Making winner's circle. Not. A. Chance. Over time, you've honed meerkat-like hyper vigilance over even the most minute changes in your body. You've learned more about what's going on below your waist than is actually reasonable. Your patchwork study of the female reproductive system would give any board-licensed reproductive endocrinologist a run for their money.

On top of everything else, your kitchen cabinets and medicine chest are teeming with remedies and supplements of all kinds − some that look shady at best, with labels written in languages you don't speak. The only thing more awe-inspiring is the maniacal, monastic devotion with which you organize and administer them all. But it's not just the diet and supplements that show how much your life has changed. It's the acupuncture, the endless parade of healers, psychics, meditations, books, exercises, holy relics, fertility idols, and other wild deviations from your sensible pre-trying-to-conceive life that demonstrate just how far you've been willing to go to bring this child home. In moments of clarity, you take a step back − as an otherwise rational and logical woman, rarely prone to flights of fancy − see what your life has become, and think, "Holy crap."

There is no question that you have the physical aspect of your journey nailed. There isn't a lotion or potion you haven't tried, a smoothie you haven't sipped, or a yoga pose you haven't twisted yourself into. You are *all in*. But nothing is working and you are worried there's something wrong at a deeper level.

OMG, Is It Me?

Where you find yourself today, with this book in your hand, is a place of fear, negativity, and doubt, hovering dangerously near exhaustion. While you have your good days, your heart has grown brittle from living in anxiety about what lies ahead. The once-enjoyable distraction of your social media feeds has become a virtual minefield of baby shower invitations, sonogram pictures, and angst-inspiring displays of everyone else's adorable baby bumps. You beat yourself up for feeling jealous, because though you are sincerely happy for other people, you just can't escape wondering, "Why them and not me? What's wrong with me?" This is only compounded by the increasing sense of isolation you feel. Annoyingly, as concerned and supportive as the people around you are, at the end of the day they have their own lives to live. You understand this, but that doesn't make it any less lonely.

After enough disappointments and failures, despite our most valiant efforts we all land on a question that by its very nature sounds the gongs of our most deep-seated insecurities: "Am *I* the reason I'm not getting pregnant?" It's impossible to ask this question without your voice getting little screechy. It's like bone grinding on bone to consider, in light of everything you've done, you somehow have a hand in your own failure. But sandwiched between the low-hanging fruit of shame and blame lies an incredibly intelligent point of inquiry, if you are willing to see it. Having coached women on six of the seven continents to success on their fertility journey, I can tell you with 100 percent certainty that your willingness to explore this question can unlock doors to your success you didn't know existed. It can empower you to change the trajectory of your fertility journey.

"Am I the reason I'm not getting pregnant" is not an accusation within our context here. It is an opportunity for awareness. It has everything to do with being smart and strategic in your approach to this journey. It's about lovingly asking yourself, "What am I not seeing? What am I overlooking? What am I blocking?" I know when you are scared, exasperated, and feeling victimized by forces outside of you that this question might piss you off. As painful as it may be at first, this is exactly the kind of question a woman committed to success on her fertility journey *must ask*. You probably ask yourself this question all the time when problem-solving at work, fueled by a huge sense of responsibility to your mission and desire to get things right. Don't your efforts to conceive warrant the same level of thoughtful scrutiny? I know having your baby is a decidedly more intimate and personal topic, but doesn't that make it even more important to ask the tough questions? How much better would you sleep tonight, if you knew that you were putting yourself on track to make sure no stone goes unturned? What if you had the unshakable confidence that comes from knowing you've covered your bases with no regret?

The Perfect Recipe for Regret: Fear, Negativity, and Doubt

The alternative, of course, would be to run from this question; stay stuck in a place of fear, negativity, and doubt; and treat these states as something you can't change. Sadly, that's what a lot of people do. They simply succumb to the idea that misery is part of the deal and get comfortable with being painfully uncomfortable. But you've got to ask what it's costing you to live your journey like that.

Fear isn't just uncomfortable; it can drastically impact the way we make decisions. Think about the last time you made a decision feeling rushed or afraid that you had no other options. I'll bet it sucked and you later regretted the choice you made. Remember the last time you settled for a choice between two undesirable options? I bet you wished you held out for a third option and stood up for having what you really wanted. I am willing to bet a pair of my stilettos that you have dozens of examples of how fear-based decisions in your life have led to "Why did I do that (again)?" regret.

Take a moment right now to think of the choices that have brought you the most pain and regret in your life. What role did fear play in those choices? Did you hold back from speaking your mind because you were afraid of being judged? Did you say yes, instead of the "no freaking way" in your heart, because you were afraid of being seen as selfish or difficult? Did you pass up a promotion or chance to work in an exotic new city because you were afraid of stepping out of your comfort zone? Did you stay in a bad relationship too long because fear convinced you "It's not so bad"? Call fear out for being the destroyer of dreams it is. You have direct, incontrovertible evidence of fear's toxicity in your life. What impact has it had on your results?

Your fertility journey is composed of thousands of decisions, big and small, that cumulatively lead to your results. It's undeniable. Your thoughts lead to your choices. Your choices drive your actions (or inactions.) Your actions directly impact your results. It logically follows that the condition precedent to getting the best possible results is the ability to make the best possible decisions. From the discussion we've had so far, it's obvious that fear is a terrible setup for that. The good news is that making great decisions that increase the likelihood of better results on this journey doesn't require clairvoyance or perfection on your part. It does, however, require clarity and a firm grasp on *the whole truth* – not just the deeply biased, short-sighted, sky-is-falling set of facts fear so readily tries to shove in our faces. With so much at stake, your decisions must be well informed for you to have any confidence in what you are doing and where you are going so you can obliterate regret. That means they simply can't be based in fear.

Fear isn't the only thing that can block your success and set you up for regret. Its ugly cousins negativity and doubt add a layer of disempowering nuance that can also skew your decision-making to such a degree that you are left repeating losing patterns that fail. Even if you aren't naturally the most optimistic person in the world, you know instinctively that if you show up expecting to fail, you probably will. It's the old adage of self-fulfilling prophecy. One of the most profound risks you take in allowing negativity and doubt to bias – and therefore pollute – your decision-making on this journey is that they can sabotage your ability to strategically evaluate your prospects and therefore your opportunities. What resources, interventions, and avenues are you not seeing, and therefore squandering, because you are so caught up in negativity and doubt? How likely are you to ask for a second, third, or fourth opinion when you so readily concede your defeat? What impact are negativity and doubt having on your ability to be an effective and resourceful problem solver? What support might you be pushing away? Are you investing in treatments that really don't make sense for you or are entirely wrong for your situation, simply because you've handed your power over to someone in a white lab coat? Might you be persuaded to give up on your dream way before it's called for or can be done intelligently – without regret? It's incredible to think about how much fear, negativity, and doubt can shape your view of the world and therefore impact your decisions. Can you see how they can get in the way of your success?

Let Yet Your Answer Be *No*

Circling back to the scary question "Am I the reason I'm not getting pregnant?" I hope that based on our discussion here, you can see that this is not an indictment of you or your value as a person. Rather, we are looking at the thoughts and beliefs behind your choices and actions, which unquestionably impact your results. The point of this is to empower you, so you don't create unnecessary blocks to your success. I want you to be able to answer, "Am I the reason I'm not getting pregnant," with a resounding "no!"

Your "no" to that question is actually a massive "yes." Yes to showing up for yourself. Yes to standing up for your dreams. Yes to seizing every opportunity. Yes to a fertility journey without regret. There is unquestionable peace and confidence that comes from knowing that you are letting nothing hold you back. In a life where there are no guarantees, there is nothing more expensive than regret.

What would it be like to live the rest of your journey from a place of "yes"? Can you imagine what it would feel to know your choices are no longer poisoned by fear, negativity, and doubt? Just imagine:

- Confidently discussing your options with your doctor, *like an equal*
- Saying "no" to being bullied into negatively biased, fear-based choices
- Seeing new, resourceful solutions and opportunities for success you hadn't even considered
- Having a thoughtful, cohesive, success-oriented strategy for your journey, rather than being stuck in the myopathy of perpetual crisis mode
- Feeling peace, calm, and joy again
- Being closer to your partner than ever before
- Knowing that you can say with all of your heart that you have truly done everything you can to get pregnant and have your beautiful, healthy baby

Giving yourself the chance to lovingly ask how you might be contributing to the problem can pave the way for you to be the solution. In doing so, you can give yourself the holy grail of certainty. Certainty down to your soul that you have done everything you can, leaving no obstacles in the way of your baby. Asking this question is a way of holding fast to the desire in your heart to be a mom – not just because you are a stubborn woman, but also because it was meant for you. Yes, love. Being a mom was meant for you. Are you ready?

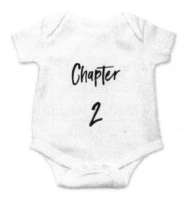

Chapter
2

Girrrrl, Been There, Done That

"Your pain is the breaking of the shell
that encloses your understanding."
— Khalil Gibran

I f at any point in reading Chapter 1 you started asking yourself, "Is she in my head?" it's not because I'm psychic. It's because I lived this journey too. While our respective paths may be a little different, the challenges, feelings, and situations that materialize have an undeniable universality that brings us together in sisterhood. The pain of struggling to conceive is unique, as unlike other "ailments," it is unquestionably shrouded in shame, judgment, and secrecy. Our fertility is an incredibly intimate topic. It doesn't just cover our clinical ability to reproduce. It treads on our self-esteem and sexuality and strikes a blow to what it means for us to be women – not because we are trapped in antiquated notions about gender. It's far more basic than that. It's about being able to do the one thing we as women are biologically equipped to do. When we are seemingly unable to do that, we can feel a kind of insecurity that reaches down to the foundational fibers of our being. It hits us where it hurts so deeply it's almost unspeakable. I've been there. While I may not be you, I get you.

Career, Love, and Motherhood?

If you asked anyone who knows me well, they'll tell you I wasn't exactly the "mommy" type. I was never the chick who daydreamed about white picket fences and playdates or reveled in the physical metamorphosis my body would undergo during pregnancy. I was quite the opposite, actually. Donning my expertly tailored, black Theory suits as I breezed in and out of the courtroom with my leopard-print Manolos clicking, you were more likely to see me with a bored, faraway look in my eyes at talk of babies than immediately dropping my case files on the floor so I could join in cooing over a picture of someone's newborn. In fact, when my colleagues at the District Attorney's Office would bring their babies in, I would pretty much flee the scene. It's not that I had any animus toward motherhood; I was just happy with my role as Mother of Chihuahuas.

This was all until my husband came into the picture. I knew deep in my soul that I had to have babies with this man. He is my soul mate. There is no question I am whole on my own, but he is unquestionably who the Universe intended for me. God definitely tossed me one heck of a break. Not only is he devastatingly handsome, but he's also five years younger. *Cha-ching!*

When we got together, I was the lead trial attorney in a specialized prosecution unit for child and adult sexual assault cases. I had built a reputation for myself as an aggressive prosecutor and advocate for victims of sex crimes. When tapped for the position, I initially recoiled from it, but it became the most satisfying work of my entire career as an attorney. Due to the type of cases I handled and my refusal to bargain cheaply, my cases rarely settled. That means I tried a lot of cases, most of which involved life sentences. My work played to my strengths, and I am not ashamed to admit that I loved being in the ring, fearlessly duking it out against perpetrators of sexual violence and abuse. At the time, my work gave me a sense of purpose. I felt powerful and in control of my destiny. I was used to working hard and earning the payoff of victory. My world seemed logical, linear, neat, and tidy, so when my husband and I decided it was time to get serious about starting our family, I figured baby making would unfold in the same way. It seemed so straightforward. I saw criminals coming into court on the regular with their broods. If they could do it, so could I, right? I recognized that on the precipice of my late thirties, I didn't have any time to waste, but I was healthy, fit, and determined. Ignorance was truly bliss.

A Wrong Turn Down the Fertility Fast Track

Excited about the future, my husband and I got to work. A few months went by without a positive pregnancy test. I didn't go into panic mode immediately, as I figured it could take a little time. My tenacity is unwavering, but when the months started piling up, I started to worry. Uncertainty didn't sit well with me, so I made the decision that I wasn't going to mess around. Like Olivia Pope, I wanted to get this situation handled. I immediately reached out to a doctor I thought could help me. Knowing nothing about how the fertility world worked, and just wanting to forge what I perceived as the shortest path to my baby, I was eager and ready to sign up for whatever came my way. Within moments of sitting down, I was bombarded with horrifying statistics and worst-case scenarios about my fertility, merely based on my age. I was a few years from the big 4-0, so this was rather shocking to me. For the first time since deciding to have a baby, I was really scared.

In retrospect, I can see that what was being presented to me was fairly preposterous. The grim picture being painted wasn't based on any thorough testing. None of the standard tests for the structural integrity of my fallopian tubes or uterus had even been done! It was entirely based on statistics and probabilities, not on any individualized assessment of me and our situation. I found myself being ushered in the direction of IVF, without really understanding if it made sense. I take full responsibility for being the kind of woman who goes full throttle when it comes to the things that matter in my life, but there wasn't a single professional around me urging me to pump the brakes and investigate any other options. From my perspective, the way it went was, "You want a baby? IVF is your only option. You got the money? One order of ill-informed IVF, coming right up!" In my mind, I figured, "Whew! Problem. Solved!"

Today, I have a lot of compassion for that version of myself, but I can't run from the fact that, as well intentioned as she was, she was in way over her head. There is no question I am responsible for my choices, but what I didn't fully appreciate was that I had completely handed my power over to a healthcare provider who, in my opinion, saw me more as chattel than as a human being who could have desperately used some level-headed guidance. I believe that in her own way, the provider was trying to help, but this exposed an utter lack of empowerment on my part, which set the tone of this entire disastrous first treatment. In my naiveté, I even believed IVF was a "sure thing." I have to shake my head at my level of ignorance. Suffice it to say, that IVF cycle was a complete and total nightmare that ended up in failure. I was devastated.

When my husband and I went to the failed cycle's "it didn't work debrief," this provider launched into a sanctimonious indictment of my egg quality and insisted that the only hope I had for ever having a baby was with the use of donor eggs. *Huh? Donor eggs? Gulp. How the heck did we get here? This was only our first attempt!* This person with a bunch of letters after her name was telling me that there was no hope of me ever having biological child of my own. No. Hope. My years as a courtroom gladiator gave me an unflappable poker face, but I was falling apart on the inside. All of the images I had created in my mind of the family my husband and I would have were eviscerated with a single sentence. My body and I hadn't just failed *me*. We had failed my husband. In that moment, all I could think was that my poor husband had picked a dud. He picked a broken-down old bird. Now what was he going to do? I went into a state of catatonic numbness.

This was by no means the first time I had ever failed in my life. I had failed on a zillion other occasions, in embarrassingly monumental ways, but this time was different. I had someone in a white lab coat with a wall plastered in degrees telling me to basically give up on the resources my own body had to offer. This felt decidedly more final than any other failure I had experienced. I hated failing.

This stirred the kraken of rebellion in me. Still shaken from the news, I found solace in the notion that there'd never been a fight I'd backed down from in my life and I wasn't about to start now. It brings a smile to my face to think of that spirit within me, not just because she's awesome, but because she really had no clue what was headed her way. I immediately began compiling a dossier of information about other fertility clinics within a few hours of me. I scoured the internet for information about what I *should* do and where I *should* go. I had heard through the grapevine that there were other women in my office who had "help" having their babies, but it wasn't anything anyone spoke of openly. So I went into full-on sleuth mode and began obliquely gathering as much information as I could. This made me feel infinitely better, because it seemed like I was moving forward, leaving the fetid stink of my failure behind. Within hours I had booked myself in with a new clinic. *Next!*

Horrified that I had done IVF without having the structural integrity of my uterus, fallopian tubes, and ovaries tested, my new clinic had me thoroughly checked out and found that everything looked great. My labs came back within normal range. On that basis, my new team took a more measured and conservative approach, starting us off with a few rounds of intrauterine insemination. I was excited, because it seemed like we had reason to hope. But as each round failed, I felt my hope fading, haunted by the earlier provider's words. I was terrorized that she could some-how have been right all along. I imagined her, sitting smug in her office, head thrown back, cackling, "Who do you think you are? I told you so! You are almost forty!" That is the exact moment when what I refer to as my Fertility Journey Psychosis set in.

And So It Begins...Fertility Journey Psychosis

The trial tactician in me came out, and I decided that if we were going to have to go back down the IVF road, we weren't going to do it without getting all of our ducks in a row. I tapped back into the fertility gossip network at my office and discovered that some women had gone to do this mysterious thing called acupuncture to help them get pregnant. *Like, the thing with needles?* I didn't know anything about it, but that wasn't going to stop me. As far as I was concerned, the "weirder" the better. I immediately flung myself into a sort of religious fervor when it came to my fertility. There was no way I was going to leave any stone unturned. I set my sights on being a shining star of fertility perfection. I came home from my first acupuncture appointment with hundreds of dollars in herbs, strange mushroom drinks, and a fist full of moxa sticks. I wasn't taking any chances. With my food guidelines based on traditional Chinese medicine, I immediately purged my kitchen of gluten, dairy, wine, and anything that brought me the slightest measure of epicurean pleasure. I was going straight joy-free for this baby! I started freaking out over the color and texture of my tongue. I even began tracking my menstrual cycle with the precision of a lunar landing.

On the advice of my doctor of Chinese medicine, I also dragged my butt down to San Francisco's Chinatown on a scavenger hunt to find the exact poultry shop that carried a specific breed of black chicken. Why? Because from that point on I was to boil one per week, to improve my fertility. Yes ma'am, you read that right. I was boiling freshly slaughtered black chickens, with heads and feet still attached, all in the name of bringing my baby home. It all seemed perfectly reasonable to me at the time, despite the fact that the only contact I had previously had with chicken was when it was neatly packaged in a foam tray and safely covered in plastic wrap. This chicken? Not so much. In my suit and Manolos, I clicked my heels back to my car with the still-warm body of a murdered black chicken, hastily wrapped in a secondhand plastic bag, which was dripping. As I saw the chicken's eyes staring back at me from the passenger seat, I kept telling myself, "I'm doing this for my baby, I'm doing this for my baby." The first time my husband came home to find a steaming cauldron on our cook top with a black chicken inside, claws peeking out, he couldn't help but ask if I had lost my mind. From my hunched position over the pot, I turned and hissed, "This is for our baby!" Seeing enough, he nodded, said, "Well, okay then," walked backward out of the kitchen, and fled to safety. I meticulously placed mirrors around our house and made sure the lids of our toilets remained securely in the down position, so as to avoid poor fertility feng shui. Can't risk letting our toilet seats mess with my fertility!

When I think back to acupuncture, herbs, stinky moxa sticks, and black chickens, it all seems pretty tame compared to the other things my fertility psychosis drove me to do, because when our next round of IVF failed, I only ratcheted things up from there. I hired medical intuitives to scan my body for any possible explanation in this life or in lives past for why I wasn't conceiving. I started taking daily medicinal baths in a cocktail of Epsom salt, borax, and hydrogen peroxide to rid myself bad ju-ju that could be lurking beneath my skin. I started putting castor oil packs on my abdomen, for fear that there could be some latent issue with my uterus that no hysterosalpingogram could catch. I did fertility yoga. I went for weekly Mayan abdominal massage. I stopped wearing high heels for fear that they were tilting my uterus the wrong way and robbing me of any chance to conceive. Even though I was terrible at it, I did fertility meditations until my eyes crossed. I avoided cold food at any cost, for fear it would make my uterus too cold for my embryos. I even started steaming my vagina with a special tea handcrafted by "wise women" by the light of a full moon! Vagina tea. I even tucked a Senegalese fertility idol under our bed for luck, even though we were led to believe that natural conception was about as likely as a lightning strike to the head. I had to cover my bases! My husband, a man who has more in common with the American sniper than a Buddhist monk, is incredibly patient, but we both knew we had come close to the edge of reason when I dragged him to a remote part of the Bay Area to stand for six hours in line as we waited to get a hug and blessing from a traveling saint. That was the point when I had to do some serious personal reflection, because none of this stuff was working. My IVF cycles and frozen embryo transfers continued to fail. It had been years since my husband and I had a proper vacation. We were devoting all of our time, money, and emotional resources to getting pregnant, but we remained empty-handed.

Am I the Reason for All of This?

When I took a step back from treatments, diets, lotions, potions, practices, and the fertility insanity that became my life, my mind began to creep over to a dark question that I could no longer avoid. "Am I the reason I'm not getting pregnant? Is there something about me personally that is sabotaging my chances of having this baby I so desperately want?" Exhausted from living with such singular, intense focus on this one thing to no apparent avail, on top of taking increasingly complex cases to trial at work, and on the heels of another failed round of IVF, I hit rock bottom. I started looking around the landscape of my life. I had done everything everyone had told me to do. My diet was the picture of fertility perfection. I was following with the precision of an Olympic athlete the obstacle course of practices that were literally taking hours a day to complete. I cried as I asked myself, "What more can I possibly do?" Then it dawned on me. I had been doing everything I possibly could to make my body a temple of fertility perfection, but I was doing nothing about what was going on in my mind. What was going on *there* was toxic. There was a gaping hole in my fertility strategy, and it was hiding in plain sight.

With the harsh clarity one can receive only through the upheaval of heartbreak, I could see that the one thing that was unclean, the one thing that was not healthy, the one thing out of alignment was my mindset. I was utterly neglecting the fear, negativity, doubt, shame, and bitterness that were polluting my life. Even though I had been doing all of these crazy things to get pregnant, there was part of me, deep down, that doubted anything would work. My entire approach to my fertility was based on fear. I chased after every possible remedy because I was afraid nothing would work for me and I would end up childless and alone. I worried that maybe all of this was happening because I had asked for too much. I was greedy. I was paying the price for waiting for the right man and the hubris of wanting it all – a career and a family. A recovering Catholic, I was afraid that God was finally trying to put me in check for my countless sins. Was I unworthy? The fear was paralyzing. I remember alternative healers urging me to be aware of the power of my thoughts and beliefs, but I'd politely smile, and think, "Yeah, yeah, hippie. Just work your magic and let's get on with it." From rock bottom, I could finally see the logic. Does it make any sense to receive state-of-the-art medical treatment, eat a sparklingly clean diet, and do every alternative approach you can get your hands on when, you don't believe things will work out for you?

I had to take a long, hard look at myself. The truth was, I was living by everyone else's rules on this journey, not my own. I was beating myself up with an impossible standard of perfection. I was using measures of success that were utterly inapplicable to the miracle of life. I was comparing myself to and judging others relentlessly, which always left me the loser. I had porous boundaries with friends and family that kept me settling for treatment that was less than I deserved. I was so focused on taking care of my body for the purpose of getting pregnant that I forgot to take care of me, Rosanne. I completely lost touch with the softness of my femininity. I had starved myself spiritually and made my connection to God and the Universe a form of superstition. It became obvious to me that until I could bring 100 percent of myself to this journey, mind and body, my strategy was flawed. I couldn't live with the idea that I could somehow be sabotaging myself in some way. At this point, I had tried everything else, so what did I have to lose?

The Method That Helped Manifest Miracles

I started reading everything I could get my hands on about mindset and the mind-body connection. I sought out coaches to guide me. The more I learned, the more excited I got. I began to see the correlation between my thoughts and actions, and therefore my results. I could see negative, self-defeating patterns scattered throughout my life. Obviously it wasn't all bad, as I was educated, professional, gainfully employed, and married to the love of my life. But the beliefs and skills that had gotten me that far clearly weren't getting me to my son. Results don't lie. I made the decision that there was no way I was going to come to the end of my fertility journey with any regret. I had done everything I could to take care of my body; now it was time to clean up the mess in my mind. I got down to business and began changing what I thought and believed about myself, my body, my connection with God, and my purpose in this life. The results were nothing short of miraculous. This is the exact process I will teach you in this book.

Within a matter of weeks, I felt lighter than I had in years. Instead of torturing myself with everything that was wrong with me, I could see what was right. I remember my husband commenting that something seemed different about me. When I looked at myself in the mirror, I no longer saw a woman plagued by failure. I could now see a woman so committed to a dream that she would not be defined by failure. I saw a woman who deserved to be happy. I saw a woman who was an incredible wife, friend, coworker, and dog mom. I saw a woman who had worked her fingers to the bone to protect the most vulnerable in her community. I saw a woman who was worthy. I could finally see the real me.

This was the version of me that walked into our very last frozen embryo transfer, using our very last embryos. I walked into the transfer room with the feeling in my heart that I was about to receive a blessing. I had absolutely no fear – just excitement about what was possible for me, now that I had put myself back into control of my life. Two weeks later, I was pregnant for the first time, at forty. The only thing different was *me*. I did not carry that pregnancy to term, but what had changed within me was palpable. As heartbroken as I was, for the first time on my journey I saw the impact I could have when I leveraged the power of my thoughts and beliefs.

With these experiences as our backdrop, my husband and I confidently made the choice to end our fertility treatments. We didn't know how and we didn't know when, but seeing this new avenue of possibility, we knew our baby would come. What I learned from our last cycle had a profound impact on me. I decided to continue to study the power of thoughts and beliefs. I wanted to teach other women what I learned so they could be sure that they, too, were covering their bases and not letting their mindsets sabotage their efforts. I stopped all of the fertility practices I had been doing up to that point and threw myself 100 percent into studying everything I could about mindset. I am not here to say that the fertility practices I tried were bad, a waste of time, or silly. But I can say with complete certainty that without *me,* they were nothing. Ignoring what was going on inside of me – where I wanted my baby to live, grow, and thrive – was a terrible mistake, one I didn't want any other woman to make. Months later, I left my career as a prosecutor to become a coach. I completed my coaching training, hired some of the best mentors in the world, obtained national certification, and began teaching women all over the world what I had learned.

Over time, I created a simple but incredibly thorough methodology for women to know they are truly doing everything they can to get pregnant, mind and body – with no regret. I began seeing client after client get pregnant, *finally,* after diligently applying what I taught them. It was incredible to see what these women unleashed in their lives. Women who had gone through years of fertility treatments or had tried naturally with no success, started coming to me for help. The results were undeniable.

Endometriosis? Pregnant.

PCOS? Pregnant.

Premature ovarian failure? Pregnant.

Uterine fibroids? Pregnant.

Advanced maternal age? Pregnant.

Repeat donor egg failures? Pregnant.

Recurrent miscarriage? Pregnant and carried to term.

While I am known to dance, shout, revel in, and pop a bottle of champagne for (not with!) my clients as they celebrate their baby-making success stories, nothing was quite as sweet as celebrating *with* them when I got pregnant naturally and had my son, Asher, at the ripe "old" age of forty-three, despite years of fertility treatment failure and absolutely no reason "on paper" to believe it would happen. This is what's possible when a woman takes control of what she thinks and believes. She can bring everything she's got, no holds barred, to the most important challenge of her life. *My clients and I, along with our babies, are living proof.*

I do this work so that, if faced with the question of whether *they* are the reason they're not getting pregnant, my clients can answer, "No. I've got my bases covered."

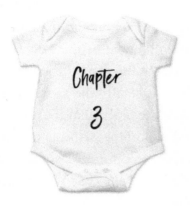

Chapter 3

I've Got Your Back, Let's Do This

"The path from dreams to success does exist.
May you have the vision to find it, the courage
to get on to it, and the perseverance to follow it."
— Kalpana Chawla

The obsessive-compulsive way in which I learned to keep records, map out processes, and look for patterns of evidence during my time as a prosecutor served me well when developing the methodology in which I teach women to increase their chances of success on their fertility journey and make it regret-proof. I remember thinking to myself on more than a few occasions, "I'm smart and fast on my feet, can stare down homicidal maniacs without blinking, and go toe to toe with some of the best lawyers in the state. Why don't I feel that confident on this journey?!" I hear women across the globe ask basically the same kind of question. The answer is that while the skills that make us awesome at what we do have served us in other aspects of our lives, they leave us woefully underprepared for the hatchet job this journey can do to our core beliefs. It shakes us to the degree where we don't know what to believe or where to turn. It feels like we have to be on the defensive from all sides, whether it be with people in white lab coats who seem to love parroting statistics, friends and family who don't really get it, employers who keep asking why we need so much time off, or the shadows lurking in our own hearts. When you consider the personal drama on top of the dramatic lifestyle changes made on this journey, it makes the prospect of looking for holes in your fertility strategy as a result of your thoughts, beliefs, and actions overwhelming. It's also quite an undertaking to try to address a problem from the thought process that helped create it. Take a deep breath, doll. I've got your back.

While I no longer practice law, the logical and linear strategy-oriented trial dog is alive and well inside of me. Being able to think on your feet under pressure is key – whether in the courtroom or on this journey. This is why simple, systematic structures are best. That is what I will teach you. My clients are busy women, at the top of their professional games, who are change makers in their fields. They don't have time to read three thousand self-help books and dabble with the DIY approach.

They want results, which is why they come to me: no sugar-coating, no BS, but lots of laughter and love. They want to be mentored by a woman who has created the results they desire, walks the talk, and has a proven track record for helping other women do the same.

This Is Journey-Tested Insider Information

What's exciting about my Fearlessly Fertile™ Methodology is you are going to be getting journey-tested, insider information. You are going to be covering your bases in ways that, tragically, most people miss. I am literally giving you the playbook of the woman who is successful on her fertility journey. While you might be tempted to skip ahead and skim for the tools, slow your roll, sister. Please. Each step is presented in this particular order for a reason. Taken out of order, they are dramatically less effective, because you haven't done the prep work in the previous steps. Be patient. The goodies are spread evenly throughout this book. Take one step at a time; you'll thank me for it.

The Roadmap to My Method

In Chapter 4, you will start by learning the genius hack for getting back on the road to fertility success, regardless of age, past "failures," and scary statistics. This chapter is really where you will have a chance to clear the decks, give your checkered fertility past the finger, and press the big red reset button. Time for a long-overdue makeover. You will love this, because what I teach in this chapter *alone* has positioned women around the world to make strategic changes on their journeys that have catapulted them toward success more quickly and more intelligently than they ever thought possible. This is your opportunity to use even the lowest points on your journey to your advantage. My clients tell me all the time that what I share in this chapter has given them a chance to *finally exhale* and get excited about their fertility again. I will share the stories of my clients Annmarie and Mirna, who applied what I teach in this chapter to their own lives and today have miracle babies because of it. Hold on tight love, this is going to turn your fertility journey upside down in the best possible way.

Chapter 5 is all about learning the secret to making decisions like an expert so you improve your chances of getting pregnant immediately and don't waste time or precious resources. *I'm serious.* You are going to learn the tantalizing truth about who's really in charge on this journey and how to get crystal clear on what will give you the confidence to make hand-wringing a thing of the past. You will also learn how to use statistics to your advantage, no matter how "bad" they look. As if that wasn't enough, you will also learn how to curate the perfect Bump Squad, so you can finally get the support you really want – even from people who you think won't "get it." Finally, you will meet my client Tracy, who beat the odds not once *but twice* because she followed my coaching and applied the principles from this chapter like the Lady Boss she is.

In Chapter 6, I will walk you through a process that will also empower you to protect your relationship with your partner, even if things in your relationship are awesome, so your journey can bring you closer together instead of quietly driving you apart. We will shine some light on the sneaky ways in which this journey can rattle even the most solid of relationships. You will also learn a really cool technique that will be like a shot of loving goodness in the arm to bring you and your partner together, even in moments when it feels like you are miles apart. My client Belinda's story will demonstrate how powerful a woman can be on this journey when she decides to have both – a great relationship *and* the family of her dreams.

In Chapter 7, you will discover an entirely new sense of power over your fertility journey. With the support of simple and fun exercises that you can use right away, you'll have the chance to see yourself, past, present, and future, in a way that can help you create the foundation for certainty in an inherently uncertain set of circumstances. Yes, certainty. Feeling out of control and not knowing which way to turn or what to do? Sister, that's about to be a thing of the past. With what you will learn here, you are going to have a trusty anchor during any storm if you pay attention and follow my lead. My client Katie will show you how women can use their creative superpowers for good on this journey, to help usher in long-awaited success.

Armed with a new sense of clarity, an articulable vision, and a tangible way to keep yourself on track, Chapter 8 is where you are going to get to the bottom of what sneaks up and gets you spinning in the fear, doubt, negativity, shame, and what-ifs that not only drive you crazy but can also set you up to unknowingly sabotage yourself on this journey. I know with all you have done up to this point to get pregnant, the thought of sabotaging yourself might have you saying, "What the heck do you mean, sabotage myself? I'm working my butt off here!" I totally get it, love, but the scary thing is we all do it. I want to help you break that cycle and recognize when self-sabotage slithers in so you can crush it and stop it from threatening to steal your dreams. Oh yeah, you know that part of you that feels like you've been stabbed in the heart when you get pregnancy announcements, baby shower invitations, see sonogram photos in your social media feed, or feel like you can't escape the sight of pregnant women? What you will learn in this chapter, when applied with commitment, will bring all of that craziness to a screeching halt. You will discover how the things that once made you want to curl up into a ball can actually be a source of excitement for you – *imagine that!* The stories of my clients Helen and Jennifer will inspire you to face the darkness on this journey with bold, new light.

In Chapter 9, we will get to know the part of you that you can tap into who knows exactly what to do, at the exact right time, and is – no exaggeration – *absolutely unstoppable.* As you read these words, she's in there, watching and waiting. I know that sounds nuts, but you've got to trust me on this one. This part of you is going to fuel your ability to move past your blocks and see solutions where there appear to be none and will break the chains that bind you to the pain weighing you down from the past. You will speak your desires with a level of clarity and precision you may not have known before so they can manifest with ease. You'll get reacquainted with parts of yourself you may have long forgotten that may hold the key to improving your fertility strategy in ways you may not have thought about, and you will feel incredible. My clients Lucy and Melissa are prime examples of women who learned to harness this power and beat mind-blowing odds in the process.

Before introducing you to innovative, fun, and wildly effective practices that will feed the fearlessness within you, in Chapter 10 I am going to help you mend your relationship with something that every woman on the fertility journey must have: faith. It comes in many forms and is called many things, but you aren't likely to find a woman who made it to the end of her fertility journey with her baby in hand who didn't have it. Whether she put it in medicine, people or something higher, she had faith. This indispensable relationship transcends any other, and when you've got it, you'll never feel alone again. I can't wait to share the stories of my clients Kate and Rose to bring this step in my process to life.

With all of the pieces of my methodology in place and after you have done the groundwork, I will share a tool kit that will help you break down the blocks, lift you above the noise, feel the confidence you deserve, and finally have the peace you crave so you can do a bold, sexy strut down the path to your baby with no regret.

Work the Method, Your Baby Is Worth It.

These may sound like a lot of lofty promises, but my clients and I are proof of what's possible when you make the commitment to live and implement what I will teach you over the next ten chapters. You may feel like this is going to be a lot of work. I'm not going to lie, it's definitely going to require your time and energy, but isn't your baby worth it? If what you are doing right now isn't working, like any smart woman you must reevaluate your strategy. Based on reading the last two chapters, you've got to ask if what you think and believe is getting in the way. This is *your* fertility journey. You can choose to live it in any way you choose. I'm offering you a chance to live it like the woman you were born to be, so you can be the mom you were meant to be.

Women from the United Kingdom to Saudi Arabia, New Zealand to Brazil, and Asia to the United States have told me that what I teach was the most powerful and transformational work they had ever done in the name of the covering their bases on this journey and that the ripple effect in their lives was nothing short of incredible. Join them.

As we begin this journey together, you are well-advised to have a journal for taking notes, jotting down ideas or questions, and memorializing the "aha moments" you will undoubtedly have. Give yourself a chance to read through the chapters and actually do the exercises contained within them. Each has been placed intentionally, so like I said before, please resist the temptation to skip ahead – doing so denies you the chance to approach the next subject with the awareness that will really make what is presented next click.

Lastly, there may be some things I present here that get you thinking, things like:

"I've heard this before."

"What the heck does this have to do with me getting pregnant?"

"This is really painful. Is Rosanne trying to make me cry?"

I get it. There were some things my own mentors and the people who served as my teachers on my own fertility journey shared that didn't make sense at the time, made me question their sanity, or made me laugh out loud. But I knew they loved me and wanted me to be successful, so I gave them a try. I am asking you to do the same. When your trust has worn thin, I know that may be a big ask. But I can tell you, it's worth it. Whenever I look into my son's eyes, I can see it all come together. Let's do this, love.

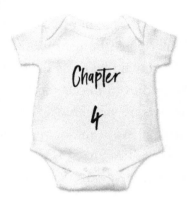

Chapter 4

The Reset

*"If you change the way
you look at things, the
things you look at change."*
— Wayne Dyer

O ne of the biggest mistakes we make on this journey is *not* doing what I am about to teach you in this first step. It seems that as soon as fertility becomes an "issue," we have to address in our lives, we immediately go into overdrive-attack mode to conquer and defeat it – particularly before anyone has a chance to notice we are struggling. We push, push, push – treatment after treatment and then a mad dash for the next healer or supplement that can promise us the baby bliss we desire. We treat this journey like any other problem, project, or pursuit we've had in our lives. Why not? Our lovably type A, control-freaky perfectionism has served us beautifully in our professional lives. It makes us the go-to people at work, among our friends, and even in our families. Everyone knows we get things done. We are women who aren't afraid of putting in the effort to get what we want. While there is no disputing how amazing these qualities are, it's a recipe for misery, frustration, and failure when you are trying to get pregnant. I bet you're already feeling it.

New Challenge, New Approach

Unlike the degrees you've earned, the professional achievements you've attained, or any other win you've experienced in your life, the reality is when it comes to having your baby, there's no direct correlation between how "hard" you work and the ultimate outcome. Even worse? We have zero control over the timeline. For the woman who is used to killing it in her life and profession, this reality is maddening. Every month that passes without a pregnancy and every treatment cycle that goes south gets chalked up as another *failure*. Yikes. The worst F-word of them all. Let's be honest, you aren't conceited, but failing is for other people, not you. I am willing to make the educated guess that you've never worked so hard and "failed" this much in your life. It's humbling and frankly, it's downright disorienting, because you think to yourself, "Where do I go from here? I am doing everything I can and nothing is working!" Lucky for you, I'm going to teach you exactly where to go from here. I've got your back.

The View from Thirty-Six Thousand Feet

Think back to the last time you were up in a plane. Do you remember what it was like to look out the window and see for what seemed like thousands of miles? Think of how you could quietly observe the landscape and see things that you've never seen before: perhaps incredible natural designs in the Earth or a seemingly-endless blue ocean. From a cruising altitude of thirty-six thousand feet, the noise from the ground, where your everyday life resides, is silenced. Looking out the window out onto the expanse of the sky makes you and your life seem relatively minuscule. You can see from a completely different perspective – anticipating what's ahead and finding a new appreciation for what's on the ground. That's what we are about to do in the context of your fertility journey.

As we get started, however, here are the ground rules. Toss judgment out the window. This is about giving yourself a chance to see things in a new way. In order to make strategic adjustments to your approach on this journey so you can have the peace that comes from knowing you are truly doing everything you can to be successful, you must think and do things differently. As the old saying goes, you can't keep doing the same thing over and over again and expect different results. If you have been ruthlessly judgmental with yourself up to this point, let that nonsense go. Now is not the time. We will deal with that in another chapter. Right now, your only job is to give yourself a chance to see the truth so that you can find your path to success.

I want you to imagine yourself sitting in a gorgeous first-class seat on a plane, with perfectly safe, clear glass sides that allow you to have an unobstructed view of everything behind, below, above, in front of, and all around you. (Don't forget to ask the flight attendant for a glass of champagne if you want it.) Imagine yourself taxiing down a runway as the captain announces your destination is Motherhood. Give yourself a chance to feel some excitement. As you take off, look down and see that the ground below is made up of scenes from your fertility journey thus far. You know what it's like to be on the ground, living that reality, but now you have the chance to see those things in a whole new way.

When you look at where you have been on this journey from thirty-six thousand feet, what do you notice? See the very beginning of your journey. How does it look from this altitude? What do you notice about yourself? What did you learn? Are there things you would do differently? Again, this isn't about blame or judgment, just notice.

Now, take a look at where you are today. High above the noise, pressure, and craziness, what do you see? See the complete landscape of where you are on your journey, as you live it *today*. Just observe. Notice how you feel as you take a look. Do you notice any sensations in your body? Are there thoughts that come up? Allow yourself to be present with the present circumstances on your journey today.

Last, from this cruising altitude, I invite you to look ahead. What do you see ahead for yourself on this journey? Kick the judgments aside and just get a sense of where you are headed next. Notice how what you see makes you feel. Are there any thoughts that have popped up as you consider what may lie ahead?

Taking the time to do the exercise of looking at where you've been, where you are today, and looking ahead has the power to change the trajectory of your fertility journey forever. This is a chance for you to take an honest look and see things for what they really are – with the inherent perspective that comes from some distance, even if it is imagined. More often than not, we get so mired in the insanity, pain, and frustration on this journey that every twist and turn seems hideously negative. When we give ourselves a chance to see it from a different perspective, we give ourselves a chance to see a path we might not have otherwise considered or even seen!

Move Forward, Lessons in Hand

What are the lessons you want to harvest from what you saw at thirty-six thousand feet? Sometimes despite our best efforts, things go sideways on this journey. Things that look so perfect can end up going so wrong we are left speechless. That's real and there's no point in denying it. Being real about things that sucked isn't about beating ourselves up or endlessly reliving our pain, it's simply about taking the lessons where we can. Whether we care to admit it or not, failures are simply a nudge in the right direction. Failure isn't final, unless of course we make it so. On a flight between San Francisco and Honolulu, a plane will take off and make thousands of tiny course corrections to account for weather, traffic, and other conditions. Having to course correct is not failure; it's simply part of getting to our destination. Likening failure to a trip to Hawaii is downright revolutionary. Try it.

Take out a pen, grab your journal or a piece of paper, and list the five most important lessons you have learned from your experience on this journey so far:

1. _____

2. _____

3. _____

4. _____

5. _____

What do you notice about this list of lessons? Are there common themes? How might you be able to use these lessons to support your success moving forward? Asking these additional questions will give you the chance to synthesize these lessons and yield priceless information on which to support future empowered decision-making. In case you need the reminder – don't use this as an opportunity to beat yourself up. You've done enough of that. Use this killer intelligence to lift you up!

Celebrate What You Did Right

Now that you've had a chance to get some perspective, let's do something we almost never do on this journey: *celebrate*. You might be thinking to yourself, "What the devil do I have to celebrate? I've been doing nothing but failing! I will hold off on celebrating till my baby gets here, thank you very much!" While I get that you may feel that way, the reality is it's counterproductive BS. Remember your view from thirty-six thousand feet. I bet from that view you could see there were plenty of things you actually did right. *Imagine that.* Maybe it was leaving a fertility clinic that didn't seem to believe in you. Perhaps it was finally getting yourself to an acupuncturist, even though at first it seemed like pseudo-scientific witchcraft. You might even want to celebrate having a closer relationship with your partner since starting this journey. Those are wins, baby!

I know you are used to hitting things out of the park and these "wins" may seem like they are a "given," but when you are on a journey of unknown duration, with uncertainty everywhere, you've got to find a way to celebrate or you won't have the stamina to keep moving forward. While it may seem like a conciliatory participation-prize, gratuitous celebration is actually a critical aspect of your success on this journey. If you don't find something to celebrate along the way, you risk starving yourself of precious joy. In turn, that can cause you to give up on your dream way too soon, or lead you to make crappy decisions from a place of despondence that will put you on a crash course to catastrophic failure. If you want to beat the odds, you can't afford to do that. You've got to be smarter.

With that in mind, I invite you to list twenty things that you did right:

1. _____

2. _____

3. _____

4. _____

5. _____

6. _____

7. _____

8. _____

9. _____

10. _____

11. _____

12. _____

13. _____

14. _____

15. _____

16. _____

17. _____

18. _____

19. _____

20. _____

Struggling to come up with twenty? Dig deeper. I don't care if you have to celebrate getting to your appointments on time or organizing your myriad supplements like a champ. Those are wins. Use that critical eye of yours to find the wins. Be generous with yourself.

By celebrating the wins, you are able to see that not everything on your journey has been a total and complete disaster. Celebrating your wins is about intellectual honesty. Most of the time we focus on how this chapter in our lives is an utter dumpster fire, when in truth, it's not. Focusing only on the negative gives you a myopic view of reality that will dupe you into making decisions from fear that almost always suck and lead to painful regret. When you focus only on the negative, you are essentially disregarding an entire body of facts. As a trial attorney, I can tell you that this amateur move will torpedo your case. It's easy to cast aside the incremental wins as being of lesser value than a positive pregnancy test, but that's a grave mistake. Incremental wins form your path to success. See them. Be glad for them.

If you want to position yourself for success and a fertility journey with zero regret, you've got to insist on intellectual honesty. That means seeing the complete picture – the good and the bad. My guess is that you are good at pointing out the problems; now you are building the muscle of seeing the good. The whole truth = power. The whole truth gives you the power to pivot, taking into account what's working and what's not.

Take a moment right now to look at your list of twenty wins. Do you see how powerful you are? Do you see the lengths to which you have gone to make your dream of being a mom come true? It's impressive. I know that's all in a day's work for a woman like you, but if you've learned anything in this chapter, you've got to see the value of taking a step back and saying, "*Wow*! I've done *all* of that?" Take a minute to honor all that you have done in the name of being a mom. Few people have that level of tenacity. Most people would have given up by now. Not you, precious one. Revel in that reality and use it to propel you forward. Make a copy of your list and put it in a place where you can look upon it *daily*. You will be glad for the reminder.

Your New Baseline

Now that you've had the chance to get some perspective, let's work with the information you gathered. Chances are that even though I invited you to kick judgment to the curb, as you reviewed your journey there was plenty of it. Let's be real, right? So, let's use any judgments that came up to your advantage. Here is your chance to assess where you are in your life and in the context of this journey so you can do something about it. For each category below, I want you to rate where you were at on a scale of 1 to 10. 1 = laughably lousy and 10 = amazingly awesome. There is no right or wrong way to do this exercise. You get to interpret each category for yourself – trust your instincts and just go with what feels right. This self-assessment is an opportunity to position yourself to achieve different results.

Relationship with Family and Friends:

Personal Growth and Development:

Physical Environment Home/Office:

Relationship with Partner/Romance:

Career:

Health and Fitness:

Fun and Recreation:

Finances:

Giving Back:

Spirituality:

Take a look at how you rated each category from a new, whole truth perspective. What does this tell you? Does this shed some light on areas of your life that could use some attention, as a result of your journey? If you have areas that dipped below a 5, make a note and give them priority as you move through the rest of this book. There will be powerful information throughout that will help you in address those areas of your life as you move through this journey.

Successful Women Know the Answer to This Question

Now that you have all this juicy information about where you've been, what you've learned, the fantastic things you've done, and where you stand today you are in the perfect place to take a moment and do something revolutionary for yourself. Much like celebrating, it's something we don't often do when we are knee deep in this journey. I want you to remember your *why*. Think about *why* you are on this journey. There are times when you have made yourself a lab rat. *Why?* Why are you driving all over creation, chasing after every lotion and potion you can get your hands on? Why, in spite of everything you have been through, do you keep putting one foot in front of the other? *Why?*

When you know your "why," and you let yourself feel that "why" down to the core of your being, you can find the strength and commitment to keep moving forward – regardless of what shows up along the way. Being a mom is part of your life's purpose. Own it. If you are really honest, the idea of anything less is gross. Becoming a mom isn't about vanity for you. It's about having the complete, fulfilled life you've always imagined for yourself. Claim it.

Meet Annmarie and Mirna

When I think of my beloved clients and their success stories, two in particular stand out when it comes to this first step in my Fearlessly Fertile™ Methodology, which I call the Reset. Let's start with my amazing Annmarie from Boston. She came to me on the heels of a second devastating IVF failure. Having worked her way up the ranks of one of the most prestigious management consulting firms in the world, failure is not something she did "on the regular." She had been struggling with polycystic ovarian syndrome and her treatment failures left her terrified that she would never have the family she dreamed of. Annmarie would tell you she was a little skeptical of my boisterous, slightly "California," unconventional approach to fertility, but changing what she thought and believed about herself and this journey proved to be the missing link. A recovering perfectionist, Annmarie learned to harvest the lessons and celebrate the wins on her journey. She learned to see failure as simply a nudge in the right direction, *not* a permanent state of being. Within the first sixty-five days of us working together and applying the principles I taught her (begrudgingly at times), she was pregnant with her baby boy. Shortly thereafter she bestowed on me the title "Fertility Fairy Godmother." We've continued our work, and as of this writing, she has had a second handsome baby boy! *Love. Her.*

A celebrated musician in Sao Paolo, Brazil, my darling Mirna came to me at age forty-five, determined to give herself the best possible chances for success with her very last embryo transfer, using her own egg. Bombarded with statistics about her age and grave concerns about her complicated immunological issues, she instinctively knew that if she was going to show up to this critical point in her fertility with no regret, she couldn't risk letting choices made in fear and negativity sabotage her valiant efforts. She began tending to aspects of her life that she identified as needing attention. She made smarter, strategic choices about her fertility support team. In a matter of weeks, she felt lighter, more in control, and certain she would be a mom. Just over halfway through her program with me, on Brazilian Mother's Day, Mirna found out she was pregnant. She went on to get the best Christmas present ever – her healthy, vibrant baby boy. With her statistical chances of a healthy pregnancy in the single digits, Mirna, armed with the power of her belief, beat the odds.

Your Desire Is There Because It Was Meant for You

No matter where you are at on this journey as you read this, there's something important I want you to know. As a woman who is saying *yes* to her dreams, in face of what might be a characterized as a "troubled" fertility past, you are walking among giants. Think of the people you most admire. Edison, Musk, Winfrey, Williams, Earhart. Undoubtedly, they faced incredible challenges in their own lives; perhaps they've failed hundreds, if not thousands, of times and went on to triumph. This is possible for you, too. While you might not see yourself in that light, I invite you to consider that your mission in this life, to love a child and raise an amazing human being, is a pursuit that's just as important. With what you've learned in this chapter, you can empower yourself to take control of where you are headed next. You can take a new level of ownership and agency on this journey, therefore putting yourself back into your rightful place in the driver's seat. You have a chance to no longer see yourself as a victim to uncertainty or the unknown. You know where you've been and where you are, and you can determine your path moving forward. The desire in your heart to be a mom is there because it was meant for you. You have the power to see yourself and your journey in a new light. As you can see from Annmarie and Mirna's stories, the most amazing things can happen when you dig your heels in, mama.

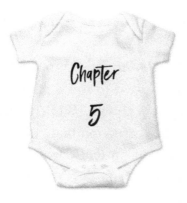

Chapter

5

#BUMPSQUAD

*"Surround yourself only with people
that are going to take you higher."*
— Oprah Winfrey

No matter how much of a boss you are in your personal or professional life, there's something about this journey that can take you from feeling like the CEO of your destiny to groveling for a windowless spot in the mailroom, just begging to take people's orders for the next coffee run. The power shift is as swift as it is virtually imperceptible. In my case, I immediately took myself out of a role of leadership on my journey and subordinated myself to someone who "knew better." While this is understandable, it was one of the biggest mistakes

I ever made – and it could have cost me my son. Let's set you up so you don't make it – or at least stop, making it – *shall we?*

Shot Caller or the Bench: It's Your Call

Have you ever stopped to think of the role you desire to have on this journey? Who will be in charge, you, or someone else? It's easy to buy the notion that "the experts know best" and put all of your faith in the letters that come after a person's name, but easy doesn't necessarily mean smart. Here's why this is so important – *even physicians* don't place all of their power in the hands of other physicians and "experts." I know this because my coaching practice is loaded with female physicians from all over the world who are at the top of their field. One of the things I consistently hear from them is how shockingly ready their patients are to relinquish their power and put the responsibility for their healing on their doctor – rather than seeing themselves as a partner in the process. Not only is this unfair to the physician, it disempowers the patient. That's a situation in which nobody wins.

I know you may be thinking, "How can I possibly be in a position of leadership on this journey? I didn't go to medical school. If I piss my doctor off, she won't help me." Your leadership isn't about being a nightmare patient. Leadership on this journey is about being the visionary – the person who knows where they want to go and assembles a team that will help them get there. Novel idea, right? Just think about that for a moment. We get so used to seeing ourselves as secondary to the physicians and experts who are helping us that we fail to see our truly integral role in this process. You are the cornerstone of your fertility journey. Your desire and your vision are what set everything in motion. At the end of the day, your doctor, acupuncturist, nutritionist, specialists, and other support all get to go home. They have their own lives. This isn't their dream, *it's yours*. That's not to say they don't care about you. That's probably not the case at all. But, let's be honest, this is *your* life. You are the one who has to live with the outcome. If you are the one who has to live with the results, why not speak your mind, have your say, and only have people on your team who enthusiastically share in your vision?

They Are Making Educated Guesses

If that doesn't shake up your view of your role on this journey, then perhaps this undeniable fact will. When it comes to the miracle of life, most experts are just guessing. Any reasonable, ethical, and, most importantly, *honest* practitioner will admit that. That's not to say that fertility experts aren't doing incredible things. Medicine, whether Western or alternative, is instrumental in miracles. The strides science of all kinds has made in supporting women in making their dreams of being moms come true is exciting. There are physicians and experts of all disciplines out there who are working tirelessly to make fertility issues a thing of the past, but there are no guarantees. Even under clinically "perfect" conditions, with "perfect embryos," there is no way of ensuring that the sperm and egg that come together will result in you moonwalking out of the Labor and Delivery wing with your baby. The "experts" are human, just like the rest of us. They make mistakes. They miss the mark. I bet you have loads of experience on this journey, which only serves to prove this point. Just think about your past few cycles. It's also true that there's so much conflicting information. For every expert who tells you to do one thing, there will be another telling you to do the exact opposite.

While you know what I'm telling you is true, there's probably a small voice inside of you shouting, "But what about the statistics? How can I challenge my doctor when the statistics are clear?" I've got plenty to say about statistics in another chapter. For right now, here's what you have to know: statistics are simply information. They are not a verdict, unless you make them so. Statistics represent a given set of observable facts, during a specific period of time, under specific, controlled conditions. They do not represent the sum total of what's possible. While they are helpful and informative, they are not law. They are not infallible. There are countless sources of scientific and anecdotal evidence of people beating incredible odds, when there was virtually no statistical probability of them doing so. Statistics can be manipulated and erroneous. Most importantly, no statistic can possibly account for *you*. You probably feel like the statistics have proven to be true, but you've got to ask yourself, if you live by statistics, are you setting yourself up to be one?

I know you might be a little discombobulated by seeing your doctors as human beings and questioning the applicability of statistics, but that's an actually an awesome thing. It means that *you*, most precious you, have just as much of a chance of being right as "they" do. It means your voice matters. Your opinion matters. Your vision matters. This realization can be a critically important turning point in your fertility journey. It will empower you to see yourself as a peer, in partnership with your physician or other fertility expert. You are both working toward the same goal. It can inspire you to more freely share potentially game changing information with your physician, instead of blowing off your intuition or observations as being irrelevant, thinking "what do I know?" While it may be contrary to the way most of us are taught to see the physicians and experts who are trying to help us, it's a powerful way to reclaim your power on this journey and ultimately share it, wisely. You are also able to take an intellectually honest view of statistics and instead of being trapped by them. Isn't spending your time looking for a way to beat the statistics way smarter than agonizing over them?

Forming Your Bump Squad

Where does a woman, who can now see "experts" as human beings and statistics as merely information, go from here? She gets down to the business of forming her Bump Squad. I will never forget when one of my clients used that term with me. I love the spirit of it. Just saying it elicits a sense of massive *yes*. Say it to yourself right now. "I'm getting my Bump Squad together!" Feel it in your bones. See yourself having a Beyoncé moment, looking fierce and unstoppable with your hair blowing in the wind. The more you allow yourself to feel that, the more incredible your Bump Squad will be. Forming your Bump Squad is all about assembling a killer team of your fertility ride-or-dies who will have your back each step of the way as you shimmy your way straight to success. Isn't that more exciting than being at the mercy of a hunched cabal of white lab coats looking down their noses as they dismiss you as too optimistic or, even more scandalous, "unrealistic"? *Eeek!*

The key to effectively forming your Bump Squad comes down to a simple but powerful question: "Does this person believe in me?" It doesn't matter what an expert's success rate may be. If they don't believe in *you* and your vision for becoming a mom, they don't make the team. Sorry. Just take a look at any relationship you've been in, friendship or romantic, to see why this is so important. You know when someone just "isn't that into you." You might have a nice dinner from time to time, but that person isn't invested. They aren't going to go the extra mile. They will likely bounce the moment things get crazy, leaving you alone to ask yourself, "What just happened?" When you are committed to leaving no stone unturned on the path to getting pregnant, you can't afford to surround yourself with people who aren't jumping for joy to be by your side. People who believe in your vision will be motivated to think outside of the box, ask smarter questions, and look for solutions others wouldn't be so inspired to seek. How much better would you feel right now as you read this if you knew every single person on your fertility team, from your family doctor, to your reproductive endocrinologist, your nutritionist, and beyond, believed in you *one hundred percent*? Now, take it to the next level and think about how much better you would feel about yourself, knowing that you didn't settle for having people on your team who are all too happy to take your money but quietly judge you or see you as a "long shot." Gross. No thanks. *Next!*

When you think about the present state of your Bump Squad, can you see where there might be some room to level up? Are you tired of getting lectures from your doctor about your age? Are you sick of hearing statistics instead of creative solutions?

Have you had enough of your questions, concerns, and values cast aside as cute but irrelevant? Anything along those lines could be indicators that you might want to change the lineup or at least have some long-overdue conversations. There are enough obstacles on this journey – you don't need them coming from inside your own team.

Since we are talking about the possibility of leveling up, let's get crazy and take a moment to think about who you would want on your dream Bump Squad. Go big or go home, right? Make a list. Are there experts in other parts of the country or around the world who you'd love to at least consult? Technology has made the world a much smaller place. There may be options you haven't considered, or ways that you could incorporate these experts' input on your journey. Be open to the possibility that you could have input from "dream" experts you might not have otherwise considered.

The People Not Wearing Lab Coats

"Does this person believe in me?" isn't just a question that applies to the experts and medical professionals on your Bump Squad. It applies to *anyone* who wants to be a part of your life right now. I mean anyone! Friends, family, coworkers, clergy, acquaintances, the person filling your prescriptions – you name it! It might make you very uncomfortable to think about applying this yardstick to people who have thus far enjoyed unfettered license to judge or comment on your choices, but remember what having a Bump Squad is all about – having the unwavering, ecstatic support of a team who will have your back each and every step of the way. There are probably many people in your life who claim to have your back, but when they hear you are *still* "trying," they offer you some well-intentioned but ill-advised crap like, "Why don't you consider adoption?" You know the truth of which I speak.

While you can see the value of applying this question to the experts you employ, when it comes to the people closest to you, it can seem like we are speeding right into a black hole. Why? We are talking about the B-word: boundaries. There are few topics laced with more angst and dread than establishing and enforcing healthy boundaries with the people you love. It doesn't matter how educated or successful you are, the notion of putting rules in place for how your relationship is going to function while you live your journey might make you want to run for the hills. However, when you take a closer look, you can see why this is so critically important.

We love to claim our decision-making is grounded in logic and reason, but the truth is, the primary motivator is emotion. We want to avoid pain. We want approval. We want to feel loved. We don't want to be left behind. Under the cloak of logic lies deeply emotional reasons for our choices. Consider the last few decisions you made about your fertility. You didn't make those choices from a place of pristine robotic detachment. You made the choices that you believed would bring you closer to your baby – you might get teary-eyed just thinking about that!

Whether we – or they – fully realize it, the people closest to us have emotional influence. This influence, when supportive, compassionate, and loving, can propel us toward our goals. On the other hand, if the people closest to us are judgmental and fearful and see the world through a lens of lack and scarcity, that influence can be deleterious to our goals. You might think to yourself that someone playing devil's advocate is a good thing. While I agree that there is value in testing the merit of your stance, there's a point when otherwise-harmless questions deteriorate into a battle over whose view of the situation is right or wrong. You know you are heading down that dark and twisted road when the person is more focused on themself than what's actually right for *you*. **Pro Tip:** people who are truly supportive of your success are more interested in what's right for you than in trying to sell you on how *they* would "do it."

While it would be ridiculous to expect that everyone close to you would unanimously understand, agree with, or make the same choices as you have on this journey, to be on your Bump Squad, they must at a bare minimum respect them. This is your life. You know what you want. Your choices are deeply personal. While there's no doubt that the people around you love you and want to help, at the end of the day, much like the fertility professionals on your squad, friends and family all get to go home and live their own lives. You have to live with you. You can't afford to let other people's expectations, values, or personal agendas knock you off course or cause you to unnecessarily miss out on options or opportunities that could support your success. This doesn't mean you don't love or care about those you decide to remove from your Bump Squad. It simply means they will have to take a time out.

The Velvet Rope Technique

To put your mind at ease when it comes to establishing boundaries with others, I want to teach you a powerful tool that has proven to be a game changer for me and my clients. I call it the Velvet Rope Technique. Remember, boundaries are essentially the rules that govern any given relationship. They are *not necessarily* twelve-foot barbed-wire electrified fences that separate us from the people we love. When it comes to boundaries, I see them as movable and flexible, like the velvet ropes you might see outside a theater. The coolest thing about these velvet ropes is that you get to place and move them at your discretion. You can use them to guide people into the inner circle of your Bump Squad, or lead them to the exit, where they can watch from the sidelines. A person's position inside or outside the ropes is determined entirely on how they interact with the boundaries you set. Your responsibility is to set the boundary. Everyone else's job is to respect it. As a grown woman who has earned the right to be in the driver's seat on her fertility journey, you alone get to decide who's in or out at any given time. The Velvet Rope Technique is an elegant way of tuning out distractions so you can keep moving ahead.

Here's how to use it:

1. Conjure up the image of a velvet rope – perhaps one you've seen in front of a club or theater.
2. Imagine who you'd like to let in and who you'd like to leave out of your journey for the time being – remembering that the ropes are easy to adjust and they are wonderfully flexible.
3. If someone has earned your trust and treats your choices with respect, then you can move the rope and allow them onto your Bump Squad. If they are *not* respecting your boundaries, well, they can just wait outside.

4. Be prepared to lovingly remind people where the ropes/boundaries are!

This may feel a bit awkward at first, and you might get some static from people who aren't used to playing by your rules, but this is your life. When you are committed to doing everything you can to get pregnant, you simply can't let other people and their judgments blind you to paths that can lead to your success. Boundaries build trust and respect – who couldn't use more of that right now?

Meet Tracy

A shining example of what happens when a woman unapologetically claims her role as leader of her fertility journey is my client and sister-from-another-mother Tracy. When Tracy came to me, she was thirty-nine and had been battling uterine fibroids for her entire adult life. She was consistently told that pregnancy, by any means, was going to be a long shot. With her history as a star athlete and female leader in the field of technology, she knew something about beating odds, but she could feel confusion and uncertainty creeping in with each withering, furrowed-brow look from her fertility doctor. Through our work together, Tracy created a crystal-clear, no-holds-barred vision for her life and her journey that reignited her resolve. She made the decision that she was going to get pregnant with her own biological child and carry that baby to term. End of story. Halfway through our first program together, on the eve of her embryo transfer, her doctor told her he didn't think the transfer would work due to the presence of a fibroid. She asked if doing the transfer would put her or her baby's health at risk. When he said, "No," she told her physician, "Do the transfer. *This will work.*" She told me her doctor gave her husband a look that said, "She's not going to back down, is she?" Tracy's husband gave the doctor a knowing nod and the transfer was done. While Tracy thoughtfully considered the opinion of her care provider, she stepped fully into her role as leader and stood by her decision. Two weeks later, she had the payoff of a lifetime. Tracy was pregnant! Her healthy baby boy was born a month before my son, Asher. Using the principles I teach, Tracy has gone on to do it again – but this time, she beat even more insane odds by *getting pregnant naturally at forty-one.* A natural pregnancy was on her heart and that's exactly what she made manifest. This is what is possible when a woman owns her vision, trusts her instincts, and demands that her Bump Squad follow her lead. *Love this amazing woman!*

Having coached women around the world to fertility success, one thing has become abundantly clear. Women who are committed to doing everything they can to get pregnant claim the role of leader on their fertility journey. As leaders, they intelligently curate their Bump Squad so it's unified in belief and vision. By doing so, each woman knows she will have the support and resources to make smart, strategic choices. Knowing her Bump Squad has her back, she's got the confidence of a woman who knows becoming a mom is simply a matter of *when.* Take yourself out of the mailroom and get your beautiful butt back into the big chair in boardroom.

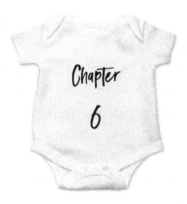

Chapter

6

Soul Mate or Cell Mate? That Is the Question.

"No road is long with good company."
— Turkish Proverb

Whether you believe in the concept of a soul mate or not, the reality is your partner is an awesome and, dare I say, *necessary* part of your fertility journey. If you are anything like I was during the most insane chapters of my fertility journey, too often your focus has drifted miles away from "awesome" and landed squarely on "necessary." Conceiving your baby is driven by relatively precise timing and biological realities. It makes sense that when you get the proverbial green light, whether it's at home or in the lab, you don't always have time to waste on pleasantries. You've got to get down to business, *now*.

Being the practical, goal-oriented person you are, you get that baby making may feel this way for a while, but when it becomes your new normal and intimacy is subordinated to necessity, that's when the relationship you had come to love and cherish starts to show the battle scars and wear and tear of this journey. It doesn't matter how in love or how solid your relationship was when you started; every couple, at some point begins to feel what I call the Cell Mate Creep.

Cell Mate Creep

You know you are in the danger zone of Cell Mate Creep when you look around your life and the fingerprints of trying to conceive are literally *everywhere* in your relationship. The carefree, fun weekends filled with hanging out together, date nights, and time with friends are virtually a thing of the past. Your free time is instead directed to seemingly endless appointments and oppressive fertility rituals that *must* be done daily, with draconian consistency. Your freewheeling days of throwing caution to the wind, showing up to a restaurant, and ordering off the menu without a thousand preliminary questions are but a distant memory. Your constricted, joy-free fertility diet has made dining out more of a chore than it's worth, because really, who wants to be the narcissistic nut job who makes even the most accommodating of restaurant staff want to quit? Yeah, me neither. More often than not, to avert the risk of traces of some verboten ingredient jeopardizing your chances at parenthood, you just stay home. What about the romantic weekend getaways or tropical vacations the two of you used to revel in? For the most part, those are gone too. With your life structured around treatment cycles or narrow windows for natural conception, who has the time for something as obtrusive as a vacation? You might be in a place where it feels like it's been years since trying to conceive wasn't dominating your conversations or your life. This is how we find ourselves looking over at our partner and thinking, "Who are we?"

During the exercise in Chapter 4 where we took a thirty-six-thousand-foot view of your journey, what, if anything, did you notice about your relationship? What's the whole truth about where it stands today? Does it feel like you and your partner are just sharing a cell while the two of you serve time (like a jail sentence), waiting for your baby? While this isn't necessarily a binary choice, it's important to take notice of your instinctive answer to that question. This isn't about judging the value or quality of your relationship. It is about becoming cognizant of the impact your fertility journey is having on your relationship so the two of you can keep moving forward toward your goal *together*.

Know What's True in Your Relationship

To assist you in the process taking an honest look at your relationship, I'm listing a few questions for you to consider. Pay close attention to your answers. Are there questions you just breeze through? Are there others that make you uncomfortable? There are no right or wrong answers. Don't waste your time trying to overthink this. Answer as best you can, from that thing in your chest called your heart. It's best if you actually write out your answers to these questions. It will cause you to dig a little deeper and gain the awareness that in a moment of conflict can save the day. **Pro Tip:** The more painfully honest you are, the more you empower yourself to do your part in keeping your relationship in the golden glow of soul mate flow.

1. In the past ninety days, how much undivided, loving attention have you given your partner?
2. How much undivided, loving attention have you received from him or her?
3. When was the last time the two of you hung out in the bliss of just being together?
4. What percentage of conversations do the two of you have related to trying to conceive?
5. Has this journey brought the two of you closer?
6. Do you feel there's more conflict between you? If so, on which topics?
7. Have ultimatums come up? Are there "nonnegotiables" that are putting the two of you at odds?
8. Are the two of you on the same page when it comes to discussing or sharing your fertility journey with the people in your life? Have you agreed on boundaries in this area?
9. Have you openly discussed the options you are willing to explore when it comes to getting pregnant? When was the last time you revisited this topic, to see if it still rings true?
10. When was the last time the two of you shared how important you are to each other?

What do your answers to these questions tell you about the true state of your relationship? We aren't looking to create problems here. It's about taking a stand for having all your bases covered, because your relationship is the foundation on which your family is built.

Meet Belinda

Deeply committed to her life's work of wildlife conservation in Kenya, Belinda came to me after a series of miscarriages at age forty-three. She was blessed with a beautiful daughter, but in her heart, she knew her family was not yet complete. The stress of the pregnancy losses began to put strain on her marriage. Belinda decided that there was no way she was going to sacrifice the family she had already built for the sake of trying to complete it. Wisely, she chose to do something revolutionary. She made the choice to *have it all* – work that feeds her soul, a deep, loving connection with her husband, and being the mom she always dreamed of being. Within weeks of studying and diligently applying the material from one of my courses, to her surprise (not mine), Belinda and her husband conceived another baby girl naturally. When Belinda reached out to share the glorious news, she shared that she wanted this pregnancy to be different – she didn't want the fear of loss to eat away at her marriage or negatively impact her eldest daughter. We quickly got to work on improving communication within her marriage and creating structures to support the foundation of this drop-dead gorgeous family she was creating. By following my coaching and asking questions similar to those above, she was not only successful in her pregnancy, she made certain her miracle baby girl was born into the happy family she deserved. A brilliant, natural leader, Belinda had the presence of mind to take care of her relationship for the long-term health of the family she treasures. Her family is so lucky to have her.

But My Relationship Is Great!

I know that when you are in a great relationship, questions like the ones I shared above may seem like a waste of time. It may seem like a "given" that when you love each other enough to want to have a baby together, your partner will be there at the end of all this, no matter what. If that's been your approach to your relationship up to this point, it's even more important for you to stop and ask the questions. Complacency can breed contempt. The fertility journey has a nasty way of digging up old hurts and insecurities we feel not only as couples, but as individuals. A struggle with fertility probably isn't something that either of you anticipated when you got together. As you've probably figured out by now, when it surfaces, it's like dropping a bomb into the center of your once-idyllic existence. While it's true that overall you've got a great relationship, you simply can't afford to take it for granted.

That being said, I will pose two additional questions based on the answers you gave earlier:

- What do you want more of from your partner but are afraid to ask for?
- What does he or she need from you that you aren't presently giving?

When you have your answers, grab your phone and schedule time to sit with your partner and discuss these two things.

You are both fantastic people, living one of the most challenging chapters of the life you will create together. Let your needs be visible to each other, without judgment. Head anger and resentment off at the pass.

Anytime we stop to consider our needs *and* the needs of our partner, we give ourselves the chance to build precious emotional capital. It's what gets us through the "lean" times in our relationships. This is huge, because no matter how conscientious the two of you are, there will undoubtedly be times when, despite your best efforts, you will let each other down. It's human. It's real. Remember that as much as this is a shared experience, it is also an incredibly personal one. Cut each other some slack. Give each other space and time to process. Don't make the mistake of turning your partner into your journal! We all have a point of maximum saturation on any given topic. Take a step back – you will thank each other for it.

Your Relationship Begins and Ends with You

What does a smart woman do with all of this valuable relationship intel? For starters, she does two simple things. First, she decides who she chooses to *be* in her relationship. Women who create incredible success in their lives consistently ask who they choose to be in any circumstance they face. At first blush, this might sound like airy-fairy coach-speak, but it's not. It's practical and powerful. It goes something like this: Will you be the woman who goes on a rampage of blame and resentment because her partner says or does the "wrong" thing, or will you be the woman who has the compassion to ask what they meant? Will you be the woman who jumps into her partner's pit of fear and negativity, or will you stay out of it, instead offering a hand to lift them up when they are ready? Choose wisely.

Next, she creates a crystal-clear vision for her relationship moving forward. Most people only have a vague idea of what they want in their relationship, but when you want to be certain you are doing everything you can to achieve fertility success, you can't afford to be like most people. You've got to be smarter. The good news is that the process of creating a vision is actually fun. Just take a few moments and think about what you really want for yourself and your partner. How do you want to feel about each other as you live each day? Do you want to fall in love all over again? I know that might sound sappy, but own it! Falling more deeply in love amid the ups and downs of your fertility journey is entirely possible – and one awesome strategy. Think about it: how emboldened might you be, knowing your partner had your back with the fervor of someone madly in love? Might you think about getting another opinion? Might you finally do that round of IVF you've been putting off? Just think about how differently you could show up. Just let your creativity flow here. Cast no possibilities aside. Once you have a vision in mind, think of at least ten actions you can take in furtherance of that vision, then get to work.

1. _____

2. _____

3. _____

4. _____

5. _____

6. _____

7. _____

8. _____

9. _____

10. _____

When All Else Fails, Make 'Em Melt

Feeling like you just don't know where to start? Let me teach you what mentor of mine calls the Butter Technique. The name is inspired by richly lavishing *real* full-fat praise on the one you love so they melt like butter. It's oh-so-good for both of you! The next time your partner is in reach, walk up and put your arms around him or her. Then, look directly into his or her eyes, and explain what a difference he or she makes in your life. There's no need for long Shakespearean monologues, contrived diatribes, or stalker-like stares. Keep it simple. Then, watch them melt. If it's been a while since you've shown this kind of emotion and vulnerability, don't be surprised if they are suspicious at first. You would be too if the romance and intimacy in your relationship has been circling the drain for a while. Be patient. Don't judge. Suspicion or disbelief is a powerful indicator that your relationship was in desperate need of some butter, baby! It might seem silly at first, but remember what I said about emotional capital. If you are struggling to even imagine doing this, take a second to remember how you felt when you first met your partner. Remember how excited you were at the prospect of spending your life with him or her. Let those memories fuel you. You want to have a baby with this person! Unhappiness in your relationship is a choice. Choose butter instead.

A Strong Relationship = A Strong Family

Your relationship with your partner is the foundation on which your family is built. Not only does a great relationship with your partner mean that the two of you can weather the storms that love to come out of nowhere on this journey, it means that when your baby arrives, the two of you can show up like the cohesive, loving parents your little miracle deserves. Don't make the mistake of taking your relationship for granted, expecting that when your baby gets here, all will be forgiven and go back to normal. That's small time, amateur nonsense. If your relationship is strained now, just wait till you have a screaming infant and both of you are in the zombie state of sleep deprivation. You'll wish you had applied the Butter Technique *liberally*. Make investments in your relationship *now*. Tell your partner how much he or she means to you. Tell your partner what a difference he or she makes in your life. Own up to your mistakes and give your partner a chance to do the same. Knowing your relationship is your soft place to fall can inspire you take the leaps that can make all the difference in the world. Do the work to take care of what you hold dear so your pursuit of family doesn't cost you your relationship.

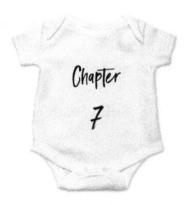

Chapter
7

It's All About You, Baby

"Your time is limited, so don't waste it living someone else's life. Don't be trapped by dogma – which is living with the results of other people's thinking. Don't let the noise of other's opinions drown out your own inner voice. And, most important have the courage to follow your heart and intuition."
— Steve Jobs

We've taken a look at where you've been on your fertility journey from thirty-six thousand feet and reminded you about why you are doing all of this in the first place. We've taken a look at your Bump Squad, so you can be sure only the most excited, got-your-back A-players are in your line up. We've even looked at your relationship, with an eye for keeping you love birds out of Cell Block 8. Now we are going to take some time to do something most women fail to do when making their way through what may be the biggest, most painful, slog of their lives – but you won't. At least, not anymore.

What I am about to teach you, in no uncertain terms, can not only change the trajectory of your fertility journey but also make an indelible mark on the rest of your life. As someone who is generally suspicious of claims like that, I get that you might have your doubts. But knowing you the way I do, seeing women in the most dire of circumstances create success on this journey and having done so myself, I am confident this lesson will be a game changer.

As educated, strong, make-it-happen women, when uncertainty about our fertility surfaced in our lives we began throwing everything we had at it. If we are honest, there are few things we wouldn't *at least consider* to bring this baby home. We've allowed ourselves to be poked, prodded, scanned, scraped, and have had strange objects inserted into our bodies. If you are anything like me, there were times when you felt more like an extra on some weird alien autopsy show than a woman trying to have a baby. Two words: saline sonogram. Can I get an amen? But that's what we do, right? Being *all in* and doing what it takes to get what you want is in your DNA. You've been that way all of your life. You study harder, go the extra mile, hang in longer, and do what most other people are too lazy or unmotivated to do. You are *all in*. Take a moment to think about all you've done in the name of having this baby. The diets. The lotions. The potions! It's impressive. Heroic even. Bravo, mama! There's no question that you've got most aspects of this journey *nailed* – but, that's also what's eating you alive. You are doing all the things you are "supposed" to do and it's still not happening. This is why, my darling, you fight back tears as you ask yourself, "Am I the reason, I'm not getting pregnant?" It takes bravery to pose that question and focus on success to answer it.

You Are Your Solution

As you are smart enough to have figured out by now, *you,* precious one, are the common denominator on this journey. You are the constant. But most people don't think in those terms. They look only to the external factors on this journey. They think in terms of physicians, treatments, medications, diet, exercise, and what's "wrong" with their bodies. They miss the pay dirt of looking at themselves. This isn't about blame, making yourself wrong, or beating yourself up. That's stupid. This is about understanding that *you* are like NASA's Mission Control on this journey. You are the epicenter. That means your thoughts, beliefs, habits, actions, and inactions all have a direct impact on your results. It's logical, linear, and undeniable. What you think and believe will determine the actions you take. Your actions influence your results. You shape your baby's launch plan. Are you starting to see how this works? Resist the temptation to throw this book across the room as you shout, "This woman who thinks she knows me is saying it's my fault!" Take a deep breath, love. I am teaching you this because I love you. We may have never met, but I love you. We are probably more alike than you think. How else would I have known that you were tempted to throw this book like an Olympic shot-putter? Just know that taking the time to take a look at yourself in the way I suggest, is one of the smartest ways to be *all in*. You can't exclude *you* from your fertility strategy. When you begin to understand yourself at a deeper level, you can see the patterns you might be repeating that can block your baby. Remember, deep down, you just want the peace that comes from knowing you are truly doing everything you can to get pregnant – leaving no stone unturned. For that reason, we can't overlook *you*. Remember, this isn't about blame. It's about becoming the woman who lets nothing stand in the way of her success – *not even herself.*

Be the Woman with a Vision for Success

How do you want to live the rest of your journey? I bet when you first started this chapter of your life, you didn't stop to ponder exactly *how* you wanted to do it. You just went straight into *do*-mode and started handling your business. No shame in that game, love. I did the same thing. While it will work in the short term, it isn't a winning strategy. It sets you up to overlook key pieces of the fertility puzzle, because you are more or less reacting instead of responding. There's a huge difference between the two. The former puts you on the defensive, the latter keeps you in a position of power. A perpetual state of reaction is not really you at your best. When the clock is ticking and you want to use your resources wisely, you've got to be smarter, so take a moment and answer the question: How do you want to live the rest of your journey?

Knowing the answer to this question will help you form a clear strategy for achieving exactly what you articulate. If you want to achieve a goal, you've got be clear about it and start with the end in mind. It's the process of reverse engineering. I bet you do this at work. When I was a prosecutor, I always started by considering what I'd want to say in my closing argument at trial, then meticulously work backward. Doing this meant I could do the ground work to ensure the admission of my most critical evidence and come up with fifteen backup plans if I needed them. This made me an assassin in the courtroom and kept me from making rookie mistakes that could sink my case and cost my victims their justice. You have the same power within you. Let that She-Devil out to play! When asked, most people are unable to precisely and concisely articulate exactly what they want. You can't afford to be in that position on this journey. It can translate to missed opportunities and time wasted. Wishy-washy confusion is a tinderbox for regret.

Grab a piece of paper, your journal, or whatever feels good to you. Set the timer on your phone for thirty minutes and start creating the vision for *how* you choose to live the rest of your journey – How do want to show up? How do you want things to be? Take a minute or two and close your eyes and let your imagination run wild, as you think of how you want to live the rest of your journey. See the images, feel the feelings. If there is a little voice within you that starts complaining about the thirty minutes, or tells you this is lame coaching BS, tell that voice its way hasn't worked, so you are trying something different. This exercise is an opportunity to take the notion of how you choose to live your journey out of an academic, ethereal plane and put it on paper where you can see it. With your vision in writing, it is far simpler to begin bridging the gap between where you are today and where you desire to be. *Commit to living your jour-*

ney in that way. Review what you wrote often. Ask yourself: Am I living with integrity to my vision? If you ever feel uncertain about a decision you are about to make, reread your vision. Then, reread it again.

Be the Woman Who Makes It Happen

Now that you know *how* you want to live the rest of your journey, exactly *who* do you have to be to support that vision? *Who* is this woman self-assuredly striding along the path to her baby, with the peace of knowing she has covered her bases? She's you, of course, just better! I mean that in the best possible way. I will teach you how to unleash her genius in your life, but we've got to finish preparing the red carpet for her arrival. It's time to think about the qualities you must embody to *be* that woman. This isn't about being someone you are not. This *is* about leveraging aspects of yourself that may have thus far gone underutilized in this part of your life. At work you are a force to be reckoned with, but on this journey, due to fear, self-doubt, and the emotional free-for-all it can be, you might show up more like Diana Prince than Wonder Woman. Totally cool. I get it *and know you can do better*. You deserve to show up to one of the biggest challenges of your life with all pistons firing. Let's do an exercise to remind you of the gifts you've got inside:

Think of three women you really admire. Put their names in the space given below. Then, list the five traits you admire most about them under their names.

Name:

1. _____

2. _____

3. _____

4. _____

5. _____

Name:

1. _____

2. _____

3. _____

4. _____

5. _____

Name:

1. _____

2. _____

3. _____

4. _____

5. _____

Look at the qualities you listed for each woman. Think about each quality carefully. Let yourself feel into those qualities. Try them on. You really know how to pick them! Now, go back to the list and cross out each woman's name and *replace it with your own.* You read that right. Replace it with your own. The people we admire are simply mirrors for the qualities we have within ourselves. They might be farther along the path than you are, but as I've heard it said, "You spot it, you got it." I know you might not feel like the women you admire right now, and that's okay. You are working on it. Know that those qualities are alive and well in you. Think of how those qualities will support you in being the woman who stands up for her desires and gives herself permission to do everything she can to bring them to fruition. Challenge yourself to *be* that woman now.

Little Girl Rediscovered

As you build the vision for your fertility journey, we have a unique opportunity to get reacquainted with a side of you that has limitless energy, knows how to rock a unicorn T-shirt like a boss, and can slip into a laughing fit like nobody's business. She's your inner Little Girl. Remember that adorable little girl with big dreams? The version of you with an active imagination, who believed anything was possible? Maybe even becoming a Spice Girl, or rescuing every injured animal on the planet? Yup, that's who I'm talking about. It may have been a while since the two of you've been in touch, but we are going to take care of that right now. Take a moment to bring to mind an image of yourself when you were about seven or eight. Think of her from the perspective of the woman you are today. The woman who would show kindness, love, and compassion for any child her age. She's so smart, sassy, and fun. Focus only on the good. Focus on what made her awesome. Give yourself a chance to remember this part of you. Getting in touch with her is an incredibly powerful way of remembering what brings you joy and what makes you uniquely you. She can be an incredible resource when things get crazy and you just need to play. This little girl is undoubtedly wise beyond her years, knows how to be an incredible friend, and is probably impressed by the woman you've become. Jot down some notes about this little girl in the spaces below. She is a great reminder of who you really are, at heart. In the end, isn't that what this journey is about – your heart?

Name five things you *love* about this little girl. *(She's you!)*

1. _____

2. _____

3. _____

4. _____

5. _____

List five things she can teach you about being the woman you choose to be on this journey.

1. _____

2. _____

3. _____

4. _____

5. _____

I bet when you opened this book, you didn't think we'd go *there*. Well, we did. Having ready access to this part of yourself will remind you to be kind and compassionate with yourself. Underneath it all, you are still that little girl with big dreams. Let her enthusiasm fuel you. As the grown up you are today, you have the strength and resources to bring those dreams to fruition. She's counting on you. Don't let her down.

Make Your Vision for Success Tangible

By now, you've probably got a lot of images and pictures floating around in your head about the way you want to live your journey and the woman you desire to be. Let's take those images out of your head and continue to put them on paper – literally. We were just talking about your inner little girl, right? Let's ask her for some help with an art project. I bet she's creative in her own unique way and would love to assist. I invite you to make yourself a vision board, representing the way *you* choose to live and the woman you desire to be. I'm sure you know generally what a vision board is and maybe you think they are hokey, *but they work.* The more we see an image of something we want, the more our appetite is whetted to get it. In fact, having the image of what you want in front of you is like putting your subconscious mind into overdrive. While we will get to the power of visualization in a later chapter, consider this a bit of an appetizer, before the main course. It will also feel fantastic to have something tangible in front of you, displaying all of the things you desire to be, do, and have.

There's no right or wrong way to create a vision board. The simplest way to go about it is to just get some foam-core board, grab a stack of magazines that interest you, get your hands on some glue and scissors, and then get to work. Let your imagination run wild. I know the perfectionist in you will be rattled by these simple instructions. Trust your instincts. Play! Cut out images and place them on your board. Then, when you are all done, put your vision board in a place where you can see it every day. Let it remind you of what you are striving for – and don't be surprised if you notice some interesting things start to happen. It's not magic. It's just how our brains are wired and what happens when we stay focused on positive possibilities.

Use Your Words to Support Your Vision

Love, I have shared a multifaceted way of laying the groundwork for living your fertility journey in a whole new way. You've dared to ask a powerful, strategic question that most people are too caught up in the chaos and noise to ask. You've engaged your creativity to reclaim parts of yourself you may have forgotten, and you have a physical representation of your vision in hand. It's pretty awesome.

It's not unusual, having taken these steps, to have snarky voices inside of you start throwing turds your way, like:

- "What does this have to do with fertility?"
- "I'm trying to get pregnant, not do some stupid art project!"
- "I've tried this crap before and it didn't work."
- "So much writing! So many questions! This is too much work."

It's totally normal. It's just your old modus operandi getting cranky about losing their parking space in your mind. Your old MO is suspicious of this version of You, with her newfangled vision and ideas for this journey. Don't worry. I'm going to teach you what to do about that in the next chapter. Rest assured that while your old MO may be making some noise, the sound of confidence, peace, joy, and knowing you are doing your best is far sweeter.

With your vision in mind, your notes from this chapter, and your vision board in hand, I challenge you to begin speaking in terms that support this new way of living. Words are powerful. Go back over your notes and think about the way you described how you choose to live your journey. Begin using those descriptors. It may feel weird, like you are making things up, but trust me on this. The more familiar you become with this lexicon, the easier it will be to actually live it. We aren't going into full-on affirmation mode at this point, but we are dipping our toes in the use of affirmative language. I know the idea of using affirmations might be a little much right now, sparking images of hippy-dippy-kumbaya drivel in your mind, so we'll take it slow. Start noticing the words you use to describe yourself, this journey, and where you are headed. Make the conscious choice to select words in alignment with the vision you created. Describe yourself as the mom-in-the-making you are. Speak of your fertility as if you *expect to expect!*

Meet Katie

My sweet Katie in Brooklyn is a super cool example of the woman who intelligently leveraged who she was "being" to achieve success on her journey. A therapist for children with special needs, she came to me at age thirty-six after enduring five "failed" fertility treatments and discovering she had a fibroid. She opted for more aggressive IVF treatments, perfected her diet, added supplements, prayed, meditated, treated her body for intestinal parasites, and did "everything" she was told to do, but her treatments continued to fail. The punches just kept coming: ectopic pregnancy, loss of a fallopian tube, miscarriages, and more fibroids. Katie would have had every reason in the book to allow her pain to consume her and give up, but in the face of so much disappointment, she made the choice to *be* the woman who succeeds. Applying the principles I teach, she gained absolute clarity about how she would show up to this challenge. She aligned with her vision and *kept choosing* to be the woman who succeeds, even when she was terrified. She even took vision boarding to a whole new level in during her last IVF transfer by creating a gorgeously lit artistic representation of her embryos. Katie walked the talk and she was rewarded with her healthy miracle pregnancy. As of this writing she is preparing to give birth. By having the guts to be the woman who succeeds before there was any success in sight, *Katie became the woman who succeeded.*

Saying Yes to Your Vision and Being "That" Woman

It should be plain as day how critical *you* are on this journey. It is from your vision that everything emanates. All of the components of your journey orbit around *you*. Realizing this, I want to reiterate something I noted earlier. Everyone else gets to go home at the end of the day. Your doctors, experts, family, friends, and coworkers? They have their own lives. They might not understand the vision you have created. They may doubt it. They may think I'm some kind of idiot preying on the dreams of women trying to conceive. That's fine. They get to do that. What matters most here is what *you* think. It's all about you, babe. This is *your* life. By creating your vision in this chapter, you have given yourself a roadmap for making it your reality. The steps might not be clear yet, but at least you have a clearer sense of your destination. Do you want to be sitting in a chair at eighty years old, reflecting on your life, wishing you had done more? Didn't think so. Take the risk. Bet on *you*. *What do you have to lose?* You already know what living in fear, doubt, and negativity feels like. Shake it up. Trust what came up for you in this chapter and give yourself the chance to be *that woman*. Say yes!

With your vision in hand and inspiration from Katie, let's get to work on clearing the blocks that threaten to get in your way. Get your cutest swimsuit on, love. We're headed to the deep end of the pool.

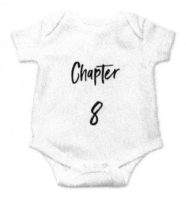

Chapter

8

Be Regret-Proof

*"Self-doubt does more to sabotage individual potential
than all external limitations put together."*
— Brian Tracy

Y ou've created an amazing vision for your fertility journey and the woman you desire to be, while living it.
Yay! At the same time, there's a part of you with her
hair standing on end shouting that it's *never* going to happen.
Chances are this is a very familiar voice, or cacophony of voices,
that you've gotten to know over the decades of your life. You
aren't the only one. Join the club. These thoughts or voices often
parade as logic and reason. They pontificate on prudence and
show up like an out-of-tune high school marching band when

you are about to take a leap outside your comfort zone. The voice of these thoughts causes you to hesitate, hem, and haw. You can count on them to warn you of even the slightest danger or impending doom. They do their best to keep you operating in a narrowly defined set of norms that have been declared safe and sound. They are what make your limbs stay close to your body when you dance (*borrrring*) and keep you from speaking your truth. *They are incredibly frustrating.* Even worse? Living solely by their lead is a fast track to *regret*.

Where Do Negative Thoughts Come From?

Simply put, they are relics from our cavemen ancestors' need to flee nasty run-ins with saber-toothed tigers. When our hairy brethren sensed danger, the information was processed by a portion of the brain called the amygdala, and the alarm was sounded. A distress signal then gets sent to the hypothalamus, and the nervous system shouts, "Peace out!" while all physical resources are directed to helping the person get the heck out of harm's way. It's an incredibly effective system. However, saber-toothed tigers have long been replaced by less visible threats, like work stress, traffic jams, arguments with people we love, worries over terrorism, the breathless insanity of the twenty-four-hour news cycle, and, of course, the fear that we might not get the things we want. Most of us never actually experience the physical threats this system was designed for, so instead the fight or flight response is applied to *perceived* threats, for which it is absolute overkill. Unchecked, this fear response can trap us in self-sabotage, negativity, and unnecessary spinning in powerlessness.

This danger-sniffing, predominantly negative inner voice is the breeding ground for what we call limiting beliefs. Also referred to as our Internal Critic, Inner Mean Girl, or Saboteur (saboteur is my personal favorite; see Henry Kimsey-House, et al., *Co-Active Coaching: The Proven Framework for Transformative Conversations at Work and in Life*, 4th ed. [London: Nicholas Brealey, 2018], 4, 149–50), its only purpose is to try to keep us safe, in the confines of the predictable homeostasis of our lives. In this chapter, we are going to carefully identify the "stories" your Saboteur tells, but for the sake of intellectual honesty, it's worth pointing out the upside of what it offers so you can make the smartest, most well-informed choices you can for yourself as you move forward.

The Seductive Coziness of Negativity

The Saboteur offers us something quite seductive: comfort. When we listen to its tales of peril and woe, we limit the risk of getting uncomfortable. It's persuasive, because getting uncomfortable is downright uncomfortable. Sometimes what the Saboteur says has merit – such as when it warns you against that last shot of tequila or strongly suggests you reevaluate whether those jeans *in fact do* give you camel toe. The point to keep in mind is that making the decision between whether to listen to the Saboteur or give that lame-o the finger comes down to your own individual discernment. You acknowledge the body of information before you and then make a choice about your direction, within the context of your vision. This is why the methodology I teach unfolds in the order it does. Once you are intimately acquainted with what you desire, you can truly and precisely identify what's getting in the way. We've checked the box of stating Saboteur's value. Now let's talk about how it can wreck your success.

Negativity Can Block Your Baby

While the Saboteur can provide you with a level of comfort, the whole truth is that it can translate to being stuck. People do crazy things in the name of staying comfortable, even when what they call "comfortable" sucks or is something no one in their right mind would choose. I saw this almost every day in the courtroom. Sometimes people crave the certainty and predictability of an objectively terrible situation to the discomfort of the unknown. Sometimes the ways in which we stay stuck are not so extreme. Instead of going back to a criminal boyfriend who kicks dogs, we do something insidiously subtle. We tell ourselves things like, "Oh, it isn't so bad," "If I do that people will think I'm crazy," or "I can't possibly spend that much on myself." Then, we wake up three years later and nothing has changed – and worst of all, *no baby*. "Comfortable" can be an incredibly dangerous place to be. In fact, on closer inspection, "comfortable" can look a heck of a lot like settling. I have compassion for this reality, but I also know there is another way. It comes down to awareness and the greatest superpower any of us has: choice.

Get to Know Your Saboteurs

Let's empower you with awareness of your Saboteurs. The first step is to get acquainted with the "stories" your Saboteur tells. Beware! The Saboteur is sneaky. It hands us an endless supply of excuses and elaborately constructed "logic and reason"-based arguments for why what we want "will never work," or why it's silly to even try. The Saboteur can even convince us that what we desire is so scary, unattainable, and laden with risk that *when you successfully sabotage yourself*, you will breathe a sigh of relief and congratulate yourself for dodging a proverbial bullet. It's unbelievably manipulative. *It has you trained.* Just like it's trained every one of us. The good news is that by exposing its influence in your life, you can do something about it. As we get ready to unearth your most self-sabotaging stories, see if any of these resonate:

- "Letting my partner know what I really need is awkward. Things won't change anyway, so I will just keep my mouth shut."
- "My family would never accept a child who wasn't genetically mine, so a donor egg, even though it feels right to me, isn't something I can consider."
- "I will never be good enough."
- "I can't possibly be happy until my baby gets here."
- "I almost hired that pink-haired, loud-mouthed fertility coach whose clients are so successful, but she told me I'd have to get *uncomfortable*. Whew! I'm glad I avoided that land mine."

See how these buggers can sound perfectly reasonable and at the same time keep you trapped repeating the same patterns that set you up for failure and mediocrity?

The Epidemic of Comparisonitis

Another way in which negative stories manifest is in something that runs rampant on the fertility journey: comparisonitis. This nasty condition occurs when you get so caught up in comparing yourself and your journey to that of others you can't see straight. With so much information online and *Lord of The Flies*–like unmoderated fertility message boards everywhere, teeming with desperation and misinformation, it doesn't take much to find yourself slipping down that slope. At the heart of comparisonitis is the green-eyed monster of jealousy. Feelings of jealousy stir a great deal of conflict within us, because while we are genuinely happy about other women's pregnancies, it causes us to look at ourselves with an unfairly critical eye. "She didn't even have to try! What's wrong with *me*???" Underneath this jealousy lies a belief that there isn't enough good to go around. Naturally, your Saboteur is all too willing to step in and scare the crap out of you, with the idea that *you* will be the only one left behind when the baby train pulls out of the station. Comparisonitis and jealousy are rooted in a sense of lack and scarcity, which simply isn't true. Opportunities to make your mom dreams come true are everywhere. You have to be the woman who looks past her Saboteurs to see them.

Tales of Terror about Age and *the Timeline*

Saboteurs get particularly ruthless when it comes to the subject of age, number of "failures," and the thing that women on this journey agonize over most: *when*. The topic of age is one particularly close to my heart, because it's one that's most perpetually propagated by people in lab coats. The notion that forty is when the bell tolls on your fertility is rife in Western culture. It's why some people look at you with almost imperceptible pity if they hear you are trying to have a baby close to forty, or over. The language used in medicine for women over the ripe "old" age of *thirty-five* (yes, you read that right, thirty-flipping-*five*) is hideously pejorative. *Advanced maternal age. Geriatric.* Nice! While women are more powerful than we have ever been, it seems like we are still in the dark ages when it comes to attitudes about waiting until later in life to start a family. If you have a Saboteur about age, here are a few things to tuck into your back pocket:

- You probably had some good reasons to hold off having a baby until now – like career goals, financial stability, and finding the right partner. Imagine that. Oh, the audacity! A woman who wants to create a great life for herself and her family? *Perish the thought.*

- In 2017, the CDC reported that while birth rates were dropping in all other age groups, for women over forty that number was on the rise. Women over forty-five? They held steady! Now, that's something to get excited about.

- Right now, as you read this book, on a planet of seven-plus billion people, there are women all over the world well into their forties giving birth to babies – whether conceived naturally or with the support of reproductive technology. Having babies over forty is *normal*. Don't let a fearmongering fertility culture tell you otherwise, mama.

Self-Sabotaging Stories about Failure

Our attitudes about "failure" have the stench of our Saboteurs all over them. Much like the way our Saboteurs eviscerate us over age, they are equally merciless when it comes to things not working out the way we planned. Our Saboteurs can rattle off "coulda, woulda, shouldas" like champs. They can also inspire us to engage in the reckless speculation that, "If it was going to happen, it would have happened by now," as if our higher education somehow garnered us the gift of clairvoyance. This is where our Saboteur can slip in the troublesome question of "When?" I will address this more in Chapter 10, but know that *when* is a Saboteur that is a combination of many of the limiting beliefs we've discussed here. It plays on our fears about time and how many "chances" we get and bullies us into questioning our worthiness. No matter what the form is that our Saboteurs take, when it comes to failure, the truth we must keep at the forefront is that failures aren't final, unless *we* make them so. Failures, like statistics, are simply information. Think back to the people you admire most – chances are, they failed a ridiculous number of times and still found a way to triumph. If you let your failures define you, instead of merely inform you, it's unlikely you'll give yourself the chance to try again. Far too often we quit on the brink of a breakthrough. As the lovable perfectionist I know you are, I understand that no matter what I say about failure, it's still going to sting. Let's go for progress, not perfection. You don't suddenly have to be best friends with failure. Just keep an open mind about it. Can you see how negative stories about failure can set you up for self-sabotage?

Meet Your Saboteurs

I bet you are starting to get the hang of spotting the sabotage! Our stories run deep, are heavily laced with conditioning from our family of origin, and have rarely been met with contradiction. Expect that they will try to hide, but make the decision it's time to flush them out.

List your top three Saboteur stories in the spaces below.

1. _____

2. _____

3. _____

What came up for you as you filled in the blanks? Did you notice any sensations in your body? Did your stories roll right onto the page, or did you have to fight tooth and nail? *By making a list of your most prevalent Saboteur stories you have just exposed the blocks that threaten to stand between you and you baby.* This list, in your hands, is like a decoder ring for missed opportunities, failure, and regret. These stories will provide an eye-opening explanation for why your dreams may remain at arm's length. Commit these stories to memory, so you can spot them as they play out in your life. Later in this book, I will teach you how stop them dead in their tracks.

Stories Block Success

Can you see how your Limiting Beliefs or Saboteurs, allowed to run wild, can create blocks to your success? If you are living according to a Saboteur story that no one but a self-obsessed, greedy brat would have an A-List Bump Squad that included the best doctor, coach, nutritionist, acupuncturist, faith healer, therapist, and energy worker she could find, can you see how that can create obstacles to success in getting pregnant? That story would systematically *block* you from doing everything you could to get pregnant. It would make some of those things "acceptable," while others were too "out there." The math here is pretty easy. You've got to ask yourself, as a result of these stories:

- What am I *not* allowing?
- What am I *not* letting myself receive?
- What opportunities am I missing?

We aren't examining your stories to make you feel bad. We're doing it to empower you. There may be part of you that's a little scared or regretful of the potential success you may have blocked, but don't beat yourself up. This process is giving you a chance to glean precious information that will support you, making sure it never happens again.

Fear-Based Decisions Suck

Another realization worth making in the context of what you've learned in this chapter is how decisions made from fear suck. I bet you can think of some decisions you've made on your journey that were largely motivated by fear, lack, or scarcity that later blew up in your face. I know I can. I have a lot of compassion for you, sister. I spent the vast majority of my journey doing the backstroke in my fear. It kept me small, invisible, and in a state of victimhood. None of that brought me my son. I'm willing to make the educated guess it isn't doing much for you either, so stop it. If you want to make sure you are doing everything you can to get pregnant, you certainly can't let fear stand in your way. If the fear-based stories of your Saboteur haven't put a baby in your arms, it's time to try a different strategy.

To further illustrate how Saboteurs can manifest in our lives, aside from just being the whispering, nagging, or rude inner voice, there are some behavior patterns that offer killer clues that a Saboteur is in the house:

- Laziness
- Procrastination
- Avoiding topics that desperately need attention
- Squandering opportunities
- Not asking for help
- Accepting unacceptable treatment from others
- Living a boring, predictable, and heartbreakingly mediocre life

Saboteurs cut us off from our infinite potential. The saber-toothed tiger is taking a dirt nap. Your life is now. Grab it by the shirt and live it with all your might. The Saboteur doesn't give a flying fig about your life's purpose – which includes being a mom. All it cares about is keeping you alive, in the confines of your comfort zone. I respectfully submit that merely existing on this journey isn't good enough – especially not for a woman like you.

The Logic of "Thoughts Become Things"

Taking in all that you have learned from this chapter, I hope that it further illustrates the impact your beliefs can have on your results. Rather than being some topic layered in mysticism or gauzy woo-woo nonsense, it's logical and linear. You can also see that while the homeostasis of our everyday lives can be a comfy-cozy blanket, if you aren't getting the result you desire, you've got to get your gorgeous self out from underneath it. Same old story = same old result. This is why it doesn't matter how much we tweak our diets or how many doctors we see or supplements we take; if we have unchecked self-sabotaging stories playing in the background, we are doomed to repeat failed patterns and get the same disappointing results. Our self-sabotaging stories literally attract disappointment to us. *Ick!* This is the Law of Attraction in full effect. Thoughts → Beliefs → Actions → Results. Simple. Elegant. Real.

When you become aware of your stories and the patterns they create and stay focused on your vision, you have the power to regret-proof not only your fertility journey but also your life. You have the ability to move past arbitrary limits that have no basis in reality for you. This gives you the foundation for freedom. It opens your field of vision to possibilities you may have otherwise ignored. You stop squandering opportunities and give yourself the chance to say your "yes." It signals a chance to start again. Think that could do some good on your path to becoming a mom? *Absolutely.*

Helen and Jennifer Slayed Their Stories and Became Miracle Moms

Helen, who runs a successful business in London, came to me at age thirty-eight because she simply could not stay pregnant. Instead of basking in the delight of positive pregnancy tests, she would sink into a place of terror, just waiting to lose her baby again. She knew expecting to fail was doing nothing to change her results, so we immediately got to work. Together we discovered her Saboteur had driven a steamroller right over her faith in her body and made her question whether she was even worthy of happiness. We started unwinding those beliefs, using the tools I teach in this book. As she walked past Buckingham Palace during one of our coaching calls, we agreed she would figuratively punch her Saboteur in the face, expect a full term pregnancy, and start acting like a "pregnant lady" from the start of her next pregnancy. Lo and behold, my stunning Helen, as strong as her name, got pregnant during her very next cycle. She followed my coaching and continued to exercise control over her Saboteur. For the *first time* on her journey, she delivered a healthy, angelic baby girl. Helen is proof of what is possible when a woman refuses to let a Saboteur block her success.

My darling Jennifer in Michigan is another example of an amazing woman who triumphed over her Saboteur stories. She came to me after doctors could give her no explanation for why she and her husband were not conceiving. She was committed to conceiving naturally and had done everything she was "supposed" to do to improve her chances, but nothing was working. She realized that while she had done everything to take care of her body, her strategy had overlooked the power of her thoughts and beliefs. When we began working together, we unearthed a Saboteur story that *she could not have what she wanted – what she really wanted was for "other people," not her.* Exposing this Saboteur story opened the floodgates for this kind and loving woman. She began to see patterns of sabotage that rocked her world. Within weeks of starting our work, for the first time in six and a half years, Jennifer was pregnant. She sent me a text with the news, and we immediately got on the phone screaming and dancing with delight like maniacs. By taking her journey back from her Saboteur and faithfully applying my method, Jennifer empowered herself to manifest a miracle.

Engaging in Some Sabotage? Clearly You're Not Alone

If you have any residual discomfort with the fact that you have probably been engaging in some level of self-sabotage on this journey and didn't even know it, you are in good company. Seeing the truth of who we really are and how we can get in our own way can be a lot to take. But here's what you must know. It isn't until we face the dark that we can fully appreciate the light. We all have baggage that is embarrassing, inconvenient, and flat-out gross. Instead of beating yourself up about it, embrace it. Let the not-so-awesome parts of who you are and your Saboteurs be generous teachers. Doing so gives you the chance to use fear and self-doubt to your advantage – yes, that's actually possible. If Helen and Jennifer did it, so can you.

Now that you faced your Saboteurs, let's get to know the part of you that can put any one of them in their place, for good.

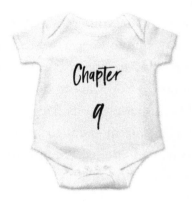

Chapter 9

She's Fearless: Get to Know Her

"Remember: we all get what we tolerate. So stop tolerating excuses within yourself, limiting beliefs of the past, or fearful states."
— Tony Robbins

I f I told you there is a power within you right now, as you read this, that is fearless and unstoppable and knows exactly how to get anything she wanted, would you believe me? There might be alarms going off in your head saying, "I'm about to be handed a steaming hot pile of motivational BS right now." If you find yourself in that place, let me remind you of that thing called a Saboteur that you learned about in Chapter 8. Remember the role it plays. When you are about to step outside your comfort zone, it shows up to keep you stuck in its self-serving program. You are reading this book because you want more for yourself on this journey. You want to do everything you can to get pregnant and hold that precious baby you daydream about. You have a choice in this moment to hang in there with me, someone who has actually defied the fertility odds, or you can listen to your Saboteur, who probably hasn't done much for you lately. The door is open. You can leave anytime you wish. But don't leave before you have the chance to tap into something that can catapult you past fear, give you certainty, and be the limitless source of unshakable confidence you crave. Do I have your attention? Good.

Put Yourself Back into Control

One of the biggest battles we face on this journey is feeling out of control. This is especially unnerving for the woman who is used to exercising a great deal of control in her life. She's got lists, spreadsheets, charts, and graphs; she does her homework; and she's prepared for anything. This is admirable and works great in our daily lives, but on this journey, it doesn't always translate directly into neat, tidy results – or success, for that matter. It leaves women like us feeling like someone else is holding the cards. It shatters the self-possessed confidence you've earned and once enjoyed. It trains us to believe, or reinforces, the idea that we have to look outside ourselves for direction. It reduces otherwise powerful women who are leaders in their fields to acting like eager puppies, looking for reassurance and guidance from others. These are treacherous waters, because *no one will ever care more about what matters to you than you.* Looking for nods or "it's going to be all rights" from others leaves you at their mercy. Your confidence, certainty, happiness, and high vibration is your responsibility. It's unfair to shirk that responsibility onto other people, and it's a virtual guarantee of misery for you. This is why you've got to get acquainted with something that exists within you, that can eliminate that scary level of dependence (which is not your jam anyway), in a matter of moments. Ready?

Discover Your Fearlessness

To use the exercise I am about to share with you to its best advantage, I encourage you to read through the steps from beginning to end twice and *then do the exercise.* This exercise is most effective when you have at least thirty minutes of time without interruption. There's no real right or wrong way to do it – except doing it half-heartedly. Make the time. Follow the instructions.

1. Find a comfortable, quiet place. Set your mobile device to silent. Advise anyone in your home, office, or wherever you might be that you are not to be disturbed for at least thirty minutes.

2. Get into a seated position and allow yourself to close your eyes as you begin to relax. Step away from the cares of the day for the time being. They will be there when you are finished.

3. Imagine a beam of light, of any color, gently projecting into the crown of your head. See it begin to move down over your head. As this light travels down over

your head, feel every part of you over which it passes begin to relax. Let the light move slowly down over your body and out of your feet, leaving light and relaxation in its gentle wake.

4. From this place of relaxation, I want you to see yourself in the most beautiful place you can possibly imagine. It can be a real place you have visited or a place entirely of your own creation. Just let your imagination run wild.

5. Notice every detail you possibly can about this place. The sights, sounds, and temperature. Notice whether you are alone, or if there are others around you.

6. This is a place where nothing can possibly go wrong, you can be who you want to be, and there is nothing to fear. This is where you will meet the part of you that is fearless, always knows what to do, knows it can have whatever it wants, has the perfect words and the perfect timing, is always put together, is never worried, finds solutions, and is 100 percent in your corner. It's super exciting.

7. Feel anticipation building within you. Wherever you happen to be in your beautiful place, get a sense that there's someone walking over to meet you.

8. In your mind's eye, see yourself turning around to meet the fearlessness within you. Take a good long look at it. What does this part of you look like? Do you recognize it? What does it feel like to be with it? If you feel like hugging this part of you, feel free to do so. You are going to have some amazing adventures together.

9. Now, have a conversation with your Inner Fearlessness. Ask this part of you to tell you what you need to know

about where you are *today* on your fertility journey. Take in the wisdom this part of you has to offer. Ask this part of you any other question you desire; *it has an answer.*

10. Next, let this part of you tell you how *it* will serve you. Let your Inner Fearlessness describe how it will remind you of how powerful you are, will always give you the right answer, and will always have your back as it leads you in the right direction.

11. Take a moment to decide how the two of you will communicate. Will there be a sign or way for you to call on it? Lastly, give this part of you a name. Know that you can come back to this beautiful place anytime you wish and receive its guidance. Now, open your eyes.

You are well advised to jot down some notes about what you saw and what you learned in this exercise. Girrrrl, you just met the part of you that isn't scared of anything, that knows all the answers, and most importantly has your back. How does it feel? I bet you have felt the presence of this part of you before but perhaps never quite knew what that was about. Now you do.

Being able to tap into your Inner Fearlessness is like having a secret weapon on your fertility journey. You don't have to share this part of yourself with anyone. It's just for you. Its only focus is you. As a grown woman, this is your chance to have an imaginary friend of sorts – it's super fun. Just imagine what it will be like to get *its* input, instead of only having the voices of your Saboteurs piping up whenever you want to make a move. What does *it* have to say about the distractions, excuses, and turds your Saboteurs throw your way? It wants to be free and powerful. It is all about your wisdom, not your fear. Keep this part of you on speed dial.

Certainty from Within, Not Without

Very few of us are taught to look within ourselves for guidance, strength, or certainty. Your Inner Fearlessness can provide you with all of that, if you give it a chance. Most of us spend our lives living in compliance with other people's rules and expectations, or spend them exhausting ourselves trying to defy them. When you connect with the part of you who knows the answers are inside of you, it opens the door to you being in Alliance. This is a state in which you get to take *your* side. You make decisions that are 100 percent in alliance with what you value and what you desire to create in this life. Indeed, you may choose to consider information offered by others, but with the help of your Inner Fearlessness, you know that any move you make is informed from within. When you have this connection, you have the power to create the Holy Grail on the fertility journey – certainty. At a time in your life when everything on the outside looks so uncertain, within you there will be the quiet confidence that no matter what heads your way, you will step up to the challenge like a queen. Certainty from within gives you the chance to make the things you say "yes" to real YESes, and the things you say "no" to, confident NOs. *It's powerful.* Besides, who has time on this journey for "maybe?"

Open the Door to Your Intuition

Another incredibly powerful reason to have this connection with your Inner Fearlessness is that it is a portal to something you might feel a bit disconnected from: your intuition. I know that this might sound like we've veered into mystical territory, but come on. You know you have it. Undoubtedly you've had a "gut" feeling that you just needed to get out of someplace, or gotten an inkling about something – you get the picture. It might not have made sense at the time, but it sure as heck did later. You may have even had intuitive "hits" about people who seemed perfectly awesome on the outside, but something kept warning you against trusting them. We've all had those moments. Most of us are conditioned to "reason away" these intuitive hits, so we get out of practice or flat-out silence them as being silly or impulsive. Now that you are aware of this awesome intuitive power inside you, don't you dare dismiss it! This doesn't mean you have to get a deck of tarot cards or trade your business suits for a caftan and crystal ball. It just means that you have a trusty resource within you that can inform your decisions. As a woman who wants to know she has done everything she can to get pregnant, I bet that feels much better than spinning in anxiety and indecision – both of which are trademark moves of your Saboteurs.

Let Fearlessness Silence Your Stories

Speaking of negative stories, as I mentioned earlier, your Inner Fearlessness knows exactly what to do with them – and it can hit them where it hurts, *fast*. But you have to summon it at the right time. A very simple explanation of how our thought processes work generally will shed light on why:

1. Our brains take in information that comes in from the outside world. For example, when you see or hear something.

2. Next, our brain immediately applies a meaning or interpretation of that thing. (This is where our Saboteurs *love* to play.)
3. Once that information has a meaning, it elicits an emotion.
4. Then, based on that emotion, we engage in some action or inaction.
5. This action or inaction then leads to a result or set of results.
6. The result then sets the cycle in motion again as it provides a new piece of "information" for us to process.

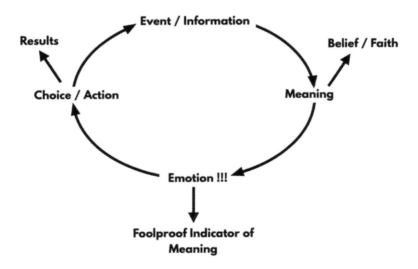

This might translate into something like this: You hear that your nemesis coworker is pregnant. Then you start feeling sick to your stomach, because you make your nemesis' pregnancy mean you are a fertility loser. Then the phone rings. You pick it up, and it's your husband asking if the two of you are still going to meet downtown for dinner. Then you snap at him (doesn't he know you are suffering right now?), and then what could have been a romantic night out turns into a double scoop of misery neither of you wants to be a part of. This is how our thoughts become "things" in our lives.

If you called on your Inner Fearlessness in Step 2 and asked for its guidance, instead of listening to your Saboteur story about what it "means" that your nemesis is pregnant, you'd be joyfully sipping wine with the love of your life at dinner. When you have your Inner Fearlessness on speed dial to help you with deciding what things "mean" in your life, you will spend more time in the fertility fast lane than broken down on the side of the road.

Forgiveness Is Freedom

Your Inner Fearlessness also comes in handy when it comes to the subject of forgiveness. Whether you've thought about it much or not, the reality is that on this journey, we've got to be ready to do a whole lot of forgiving. Forgiving the members of our Bump Squad who let us down, our coworkers who engage in gossip and speculation about why we are missing so much work, our friends and family who say stupid things, and most importantly, ourselves. You might be a master grudge holder and it might feel fiendishly awesome to make scathing remarks about the people you think have done you wrong, but forgiveness isn't about them. It's about you. It's about reclaiming your energy from people who aren't contributing to your success and pointing that precious resource back where it belongs: you.

Forgiving yourself and other people doesn't mean that what happened didn't suck or that you give anyone license to do it again, it's simply about burying the hatchet already, because you've got more important projects to focus your attention on – like baby making. You can't possibly show up 100 percent to that when 45 percent of you is worrying about what Bitter Bee said to you three weeks ago. Don't forget your Velvet Rope Tool, from Chapter 5. If certain people in your life need a time out, make the adjustments to your Velvet Rope accordingly. Forgiveness can be a hard thing at first, but remember it's for and about *you*. Forgiveness doesn't even require another person's participation. You control everything about it! (Super exciting!) There are loads of treatises on the subject of forgiveness, so if you feel the desire to dig a little deeper into it, rock on, mama. Here's a simple exercise that I like to use when I've got some forgiving to do:

1. Bust out a piece of paper or your journal and write a letter to the person, situation, or circumstance you choose to forgive. Don't forget to include yourself.
2. Hold nothing back. Rip 'em a new one. Go bananas. Air all of your grievances.
3. Thank the person, situation, or circumstance for teaching you a lesson. Name the specific lesson.
4. Write why it's time to let this go. What's it costing you to carry it around?
5. Write the words, "I forgive you."
6. Take the piece of paper or page out of your journal and get rid of it. Some people like to burn letters like this. You do whatever you like – flush it, shred it, or just throw it away.

Notice how you feel after doing this. If you are still feeling unsettled, that doesn't mean you failed the exercise. It just means what you feel probably runs deep. If you have to do this a few more times on the same subject, cool. Keep doing it until you feel free. *It will get better.* Keep asking your Inner Fearlessness for guidance. Give yourself a chance to free up your energy so you can bring 100 percent of yourself to your journey. Forgiveness is freedom.

Reclaiming Your Feminine Power

Unleashing your Inner Fearlessness can also return you to something you may have left in the dust long ago: femininity. You might have the overwhelming impulse to throw this book across the room (again), but hear me out. I'm not questioning how much of a woman you are, nor am I suggesting that you have to relegate yourself to 1950s Housewife Status. We aren't talking about gender or gender roles at all. I'm pointing to the fact that within all of us exists masculine and feminine energy. The masculine tends to be what drives us to work harder, push longer, and get things done. The feminine is the creative, spiritual, loving, maternal, and emotional side of ourselves. The feminine isn't something that is typically rewarded in the workplace or generally in our society. The feminine is often maligned as messy, unreliable, and weak. But, let me remind you, *you are trying to do the most feminine thing you can possibly do*: have a baby. Does it make any sense to try to do the most feminine thing you can possibly do in your masculine?

When I realized I was living my fertility journey "like a man," I was floored – not just because it was kind of laughable, but also because I could see how trying to do something inextricably feminine with masculine energy was setting me up to fail. As a trial attorney, I was used to operating in my masculine. Pushing, striving, and living with a "take no prisoners" attitude is what made me so good in the courtroom, but it disconnected me from all the feminine alarms that were going off within me, telling me I needed to rest, reduce my stress, and take better care of myself. I wore my burnout like a badge of honor. Why not? It had worked so well in every other aspect of my life. Except, of course when it came to making babies.

Here are some warning signs that you might be trying to get pregnant *like a man:*

- Pushing through treatment after treatment, with little to no breaks
- Ignoring the fact that you are exhausted
- Downplaying your pain because "it's just part of the deal"
- Ignoring your intuition
- Not asking for help
- Beating yourself up, because you just can't seem to do anything right
- Realizing it's been way too long since you've had a vacation

Reconnecting with your feminine energy doesn't require you to suddenly start wearing long, flowing dresses or be any less in control of your life. It's about learning to marshal your energy intelligently. There will be times when pushing through is required, but you've got to be able to hear your feminine when she's telling you to slow down. Your feminine will remind you why you are doing all of this in the first place. It's about the love in your heart. You know how to live your journey from the neck up – defaulting to what's logical and linear according to your brain. Now it's time to start incorporating the goodness found from the neck down, by considering what's in your heart and how things *feel*.

To get your ideas flowing about reconnecting with your femininity, grab a piece of paper or your journal and start brainstorming about how you can experience more of it. Do you long to take a break from trying to conceive? Would you like to start taking better care of *you* – the woman on the inside? Is it time you engaged more of your heart instead of relying entirely on what's logical? Could you use more creativity? As women, we get to be the architects of our own femininity. We don't have to follow other people's rules about what that means. Create your own definition and own it.

Lucy and Melissa Rediscovered Their Fearlessness and Beat the Odds

A high-achieving prodigy and physician from Ohio, Lucy came to me because her thirty-two-year-old body was acting more like it was in menopause than in its baby-making prime. Her colleagues in medicine had given her a *less than 10 percent chance* of ever conceiving naturally and told her the best possible option for her to get pregnant was with the use of donor eggs. Her medical training made it hard to look past the statistics and tangible "evidence," but she wasn't ready to give up on her body's own resources. With her enviably wild mass of beautiful curls as her crown, Lucy went about the business of supporting her vision of conceiving her own biological child naturally, like a queen. With my coaching, she dismantled the stories of her Saboteurs, which led to her curating a stellar Bump Squad, and committed to her success even though on paper it seemed unlikely. Lucy brought 100 percent of herself to her journey – mind and body. Then, about two months after attending one of my retreats, Lucy beat single-digit odds by *getting pregnant naturally*. As a result of becoming the woman who thinks out of the box, does not let past failures or statistics define her, and makes her own rules, Lucy learned to trust her Inner Fearlessness. As of this writing, she is gliding smoothly into her third trimester, expecting a healthy baby boy.

Melissa, an insanely funny and gifted pediatrician from California, came to me after a long history of fertility treatment failures, which even included the use of donor eggs. Like Lucy, she found it hard to look beyond the medical evidence in front of her and the dismal prognosis it painted. The pain of constantly seeing newborns with their parents in her practice only compounded her grief. Melissa longed to feel peace and confidence in her body. She had done absolutely everything she could *physically* to get pregnant – she instinctively knew the missing piece was her mind. We immediately got to work, because there was no way she was going to let negativity sabotage her chances with the embryos she had left. A few months into our work together, you guessed it! Melissa was pregnant with her adorable baby boy and absolutely rocking being the mom she was so meant to be!

What makes Lucy and Melissa's stories particularly moving is that in light of their intense professional training, they would have had *every reason* to give up, but they didn't. These brave women had the guts to believe in themselves when virtually every fiber of their intellect was trying to drag them in the opposite direction. They had to see beyond the grim, harsh reality their profession tried to force feed them. They dared to pursue their dream of motherhood from the neck down. They are living proof that mindset elevates medicine.

The truest kind of fearlessness is about using the resources within you intelligently, from tapping into the part of you that can discern real threats from the whiney nonsense of your Saboteurs, to finding certainty within and showing up to this journey as the unstoppable success you deserve to be. These resources exist in you today. You now have the tools to start calling on them at will. Give yourself the chance to let your fearlessness lead the way. Just imagine what the two of you can create.

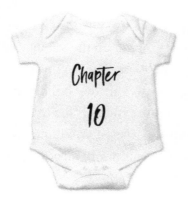

Chapter
10

Faith: Your First Resort, Not Your Last.

"Faith is taking the first step even when you don't see the whole staircase."
— Martin Luther King Jr.

Never in a thousand years would I have thought I'd write a book that would include a chapter on the subject of faith. It's a topic I struggled with, turned my back on, and, on the darkest days, mocked. I'm not exactly sure what soured me to the subject of faith. Maybe it was the fear with which it was presented to me as a child, or perhaps it was the PTSD I suffered after being dragged across the school playground by a nun who had a vice-like grip on my ear. Either way, until the last few years of my fertility journey, there would have been no way I'd be bringing up the subject of faith.

My point in going "there" with you is not to proselytize any specific set of religious or spiritual beliefs. Rather, it's an invitation for you to explore for yourself the role it can play, within the context of your fertility. Even if you think you have a reasonably good relationship with your faith, buckle up, love, I've got a few things in store for you.

Got Faith?

First things first, what is the state of your faith as you read this? Are you in a place where even reading that word made you scoff or roll your eyes, muttering, "I don't need unseen forces or superstition to bring home this baby. I can skip this chapter!" Are you angry with God/the Universe/Source, because no matter how hard you've prayed, or how fervently you've asked, it has failed to put a baby in your arms? Is there something about faith that feels fake, because you don't have any and to get some now seems hypocritical? Does this whole topic make your skin crawl? If you are wrestling with any of those notions or some version of them, I get it.

If you had asked me about faith during the vast majority of my fertility journey, I would have smiled politely and thought to myself, "How sweet. She thinks I need faith. Who needs that, when you've got medicine?" While there was part of me that was vaguely open to the idea of a higher power, whatever it may be, I have to admit I approached the subject with incredible hubris, condescension, and judgment. I had cut myself off from faith to such a degree, I saw it as self-soothing for simpletons. I bit my tongue and feigned gratitude when people would tell me they were praying for me. It seemed silly to me to waste my time on the subject of faith, because if medicine couldn't help me, nothing could. Then I hit rock bottom.

Seeing the Signs with Open Eyes

On the same day I won a guilty verdict in one of the most important cases in my career as a prosecutor, I also got the news that yet another one of my IVF cycles had failed. I remember leaning against the cold wall in my office, raging, as I fought back tears. I had done everything Western and alternative medicine told me to do. Again, I was empty-handed. *Why was I doing all of this?* Then, I went numb, again. A few days later, I was in the shower and unexpectedly a song by Darius Rucker, "True Believers," came on, and I wept. I say "unexpectedly" because there was absolutely nothing in my streaming music feed that would have included a country-ish song, much less one that included the word *God*. As Darius sung about faith, I howled like a baby. The only way I can explain it is that in that moment, as the warm water pounded against my body, bruised, bloated, and scarred from years of fertility treatments, I felt the power of what I refer to as God. For decades I struggled with that word, but there was no question in my mind that that is exactly what I felt. I made a decision in that moment that I'd follow wherever that feeling led me. I kept that experience to myself for the longest time. Back then, my husband wasn't much of a believer, and I didn't want him to suspect I had slipped in the shower, hit my head, and then woke up as some kind of spiritual zealot.

I'm sharing this with you, because what came next was nothing short of miraculous. I was wildly out of practice with prayer, so I just started asking "whomever" was "out there" to give me signs and keep me in mind. In very short order, I began noticing synchronicities that can only be described as grace showing up in my life. Loving experts, teachers, healers, and coaches, and game-changing books, movies, and signs began popping up everywhere in my life. At a time when I had absolutely no reason to – with my ridiculous history of failure, and about to hit forty – I had faith. A short time later, having transformed my thoughts and beliefs, connected with my faith, and taken full responsibility for being the woman who succeeds on this journey, *I got pregnant for the very first time.* I was grateful for that miracle, but another miracle came on its heels that blew my mind and solidified my unwavering faith that no matter what, my son was on the way: a woman from Kenya.

The Miracle from Kenya

My IVF doctor had given me a lab order to do a second beta test for HCG to confirm that my pregnancy was progressing. That happened to fall on Thanksgiving Day. I had to drive an hour to the nearest lab that was open, which ended up being a major metropolitan hospital. When I got there, I expected it to look like post-apocalyptic scene from the movie *Escape from New York*, with a waiting room full of junkies and gunshot victims. I checked in and waited. Moments later, a woman came walking down the hall and called my name. I got up and quickly followed her. She led me down a quiet hallway, away from the chaos, and opened the door to a room that, no joke, was awash with the most beautiful golden light coming through the windows from the outside. It was like I had stepped into another dimension. The woman told me that she had moved from Kenya, had only been in California for three months, and was looking forward to having her first Thanksgiving dinner. Then abruptly, her face went blank, she looked at the lab slip, and then looked at me square in the eye and said, "You need a prayer, don't you?" I was stunned.

What she could not possibly have known, because I was not a patient at that hospital, they did not have any of my history, and there was nothing indicated on my lab slip, was that the number from my first beta test was low. My treatment team was waiting with bated breath to see if the number would double, thereby indicating a progressing pregnancy. I burst into tears and said, "Yes. Yes, ma'am I do." She then took both of my hands into hers and began praying out loud for me. I thought my head was going to explode. I never imagined that I'd find myself in tears with my hands held by some woman I had never met, praying for me and my baby, in a secular hospital. You could get sued for that, right? None of my silliness stopped her. When she completed the prayer, I thanked her, she did my blood draw, she walked me out, and I never saw her again. I never even caught her name. She simply disappeared. My eyes well up every time I share that story – as they are now. There is no question in my mind that she was an angel. In a moment I needed faith most, it made a bold, undeniable appearance.

Faith Is a Relationship, a Conversation

I know that the subject of faith can be complicated and rife with contradiction, but faith on this journey, in my opinion, isn't about adherence to doctrinal purity. It's about a relationship. A relationship with something greater that put the desire in your heart to be a mom. A desire that was meant for you, as part of your life's purpose. I will never forget one of my favorite mentors saying, "Faith and fear require us to believe in something we can't see. Choose wisely." Faith is simply a way to connect with that wisdom and knowing inside of you what we talked about in Chapter 9. Faith is what bridges the gap between where you are today and where you want to be. Faith in your purpose and the vision you have for motherhood will fuel your creativity, resourcefulness, and keep you putting one foot in front of the other, in the face of setbacks and disappointments. Faith keeps your eye on the prize.

If it's been a while since you've hung out with faith, don't worry; you don't have to jump onto some parochial bandwagon. It can start as a conversation. If the idea of prayer doesn't work for you, consider it simply connecting with a higher power. You can call that meditation, as many philosophies do. Just keep an open heart and mind. The snarky side of you might be tempted to issue ludicrous challenges like, "Okay, Higher Power, I will show some faith, if you strike my boss with a bolt of lightning, right … about … now!" If you are that committed to skepticism, try again another day.

Faith as the Cornerstone of Surrender

Here's another reason to build your faith: faith is the cornerstone of surrender. If you want to end the daily agonizing about *when* and *how* your baby will get here, you must have faith, because no human being can provide you with those answers. If they could, none of us would suffer a day on this journey. Surrender is in many ways about allowing your journey to unfold, believing that the timing and events are happening *for* you, not *to* you. Surrender is quite a powerful position to be in, as it demonstrates faith in the process. It's like saying, "I may not know when, I may not know how, but I *know* my baby is coming." As a woman committed to being a mom, isn't that what you must believe in order to stay the course? Surrender isn't about giving up. It's about giving yourself a chance to lean back, exhale, and receive.

Build Faith with Gratitude

A surefire way to jump-start your faith is gratitude. It's a topic that people love to throw around, but rather than waste time on platitudes, I want to give you a chance to see it as tangible proof that something "out there" indeed has your back. Most of us grow up with notions of gratitude that are intended to make us feel small and ashamed of wanting more than we already have. How many times have you heard someone say, "Just be grateful for what you've got," as a way of knocking you down to size? What if gratitude is intended to demonstrate the abundance that is possible? What if gratitude is a way of keeping us focused on how there is a steady source of good in our lives?

Take a moment right now to think of the ten things for which you are most grateful.

1. _____

2. _____

3. _____

4. _____

5. _____

6. _____

7. _____

8. _____

9. _____

10. _____

Awesome stuff, right? You are blessed indeed. This shows you how much good has come into your life. Who's to say that's the limit? Certainly there are thousands of things you can be grateful for, so I hope you can see how much abundance there is in your life – whether you've specifically asked for it or not. When the chips are down, there's no real lack of resources, opportunities, money, or chances. They are there for the taking if you are willing to see them. With an expansive sense of gratitude, you can see there's more than enough good in the world, which means there's more than enough for you. When you get this idea in your bones, you open your heart up to receiving all that you need on this journey. If you think about it from a practical and metaphorical standpoint, conceiving is all about receiving, isn't it?

Have Faith in Your Body

Whether you believe in the Big Bang, Divine Creation, or that we all just suddenly appeared, there can be no question that we are all made up of atoms that come together to form matter. Having had your fair share of seeing cells divide in a lab, you know there is some kind of intelligence that gets the cells to do what they do. Somehow a finger knows how to heal from a cut and our bodies find a way to adapt to the conditions we are in. When we think about the magic of all of that, it's breathtaking. The human body is a symphony of complex systems coming together to make *you.* When you stop and think about that, you can see that your body is a pretty awesome thing. When was the last time you thought of yourself in that way? Your body is a demonstration of divine intelligence. It's the only body you've got! Cut it some slack. Faith can help you see that your body isn't just a meat suit that can't seem to get it together enough to give you a baby. You are the divine's highest creation. Trust it. Trust yourself.

Kate and Rose Let Faith Guide Them to Miracles

A registered nurse from the great state of Rhode Island, Kate came to me after struggling for years to conceive. She is a woman of faith but was finding it harder to believe in the face of so much disappointment. She and her husband decided against interventions such as IUI and IVF. Kate was committed to conceiving her baby naturally. She approached our coaching sessions with a beginner's heart, eager to learn and apply the lessons. She courageously challenged her fertility issues being lazily categorized as "unexplained." She began advocating for herself in bold, self-assured ways. She became the woman who was *not* leaving the Earth without her baby! Kate allowed herself to explore her femininity, reconnecting with her passion for art, and even leveling up her communication with her husband using the legendary Butter Technique (see Chapter 6). Following the steps in this process, she reignited her faith. Approximately seven months later, Kate was pregnant naturally, as she had set her mind and faith to be.

Rose, a brilliant Harvard-educated Canadian physician, came to me after suffering a series of heart-wrenching losses, ectopic pregnancy, and bumbling misdiagnoses that rattled her faith not only in medicine, but also her higher power. Rose's journey included challenges to her very identity, as concerns were raised that her heritage could be a contributing factor to her fertility issues, and experiencing bigotry in the process, due to her being part of the LGBTQ community. Rose faced gargantuan blocks on the road to her baby, but she chose her vision over her fear. Ever the star student, Rose immediately began applying the tools and strategies outlined in this book. She rebuilt her faith and empowered herself to pursue new options for bringing home her baby. Despite harrowing detours, through the blessing of egg donation and surrogacy, Rose and her amazing wife's prayers for a baby were answered. Like so many of the extraordinary women who I have had the honor of coaching, by allowing herself to *be* the woman who succeeds, Rose *became* the woman who succeeded.

Let Faith Bridge the Gap

Being a mom is part of your life's purpose. You know it was meant for you. Fuel and deepen that knowing with your faith. Let your faith be a unique expression of you. Let it be no one's business but yours. Miracles don't necessarily have to come in parting of seas or sight to the blind. It can be something as simple as a kind word, or loving people in your life showing up at the right time. Open your eyes and your heart to see your own "signs." I bet you will start seeing them everywhere. Faith is what bridges the gap between where you are today and where you want to be. We all put faith in something – medicine, Murphy's law, karma, you name it. Why not put your faith in the Universe that created you? Make faith your first resort, not your last.

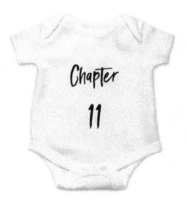

Chapter
11

The Toolbox/Making It Stick

*"The most difficult thing is the decision to act. The rest
is merely tenacity. The fears are paper tigers. You can do
anything you decide to do. You can act to change and control
your life; and the procedure, the process is its own reward."*
— Amelia Earhart

We've been on quite a journey together at this point. You've become aware of your vision and identified the "stories" that get in the way, you now know what you desire from your Bump Squad and relationships, and you've defined your brand of femininity and dusted off your faith. You have foundational building blocks to change the unconscious thought patterns that can foster fear, negativity, a sense of scarcity, lack, jealousy, isolation, and doubt, as well as their associated behaviors – which can block your success. I'm sure we've pushed a few buttons and unveiled some massive a-has. While all of that is fantastic, there's also no question in my mind that there's part of you wondering how the heck you are going to synthesize this mountain of information. I've had your back this whole way, love, and it's not going to stop now. In this chapter, I am going to teach you a series of daily practices, tools, and strategies to feed the fearlessness within you, so you can live your fertility journey from a place of empowerment, not under the constant threat of regret.

Each of the tools I am going to share with you here coincides with each step of the methodology I have unveiled in this book. These are intended to be elegant additions to your daily life and are not intended to be cumbersome or confusing. There's no way to do any of these things "wrong" per se. When in doubt, remember that these tools are intended to support you. Beware the Saboteur that may start complaining about having "one more thing to do or remember." The role of the Saboteur is to try to keep you in stasis. It wants you to stay stuck, because it's comfortable. As seductive as that might be, results don't lie. If doing things the Saboteur's way hasn't put a baby in your arms, why stick with that stagnant program?

Let me also remind you that your decision to think and do things differently on this journey will be a *daily* choice. There will be times when you feel like things are falling in place blissfully easily. There will also be times when things seem to be sliding backward and you may doubt why you even bothered with this. When either shows up, celebrate it and keep moving forward. Remember your *why*. You are challenging yourself here, because you want to be 100 percent sure you are doing everything you can to bring that precious baby home. Now is not the time to quit or get lazy. Just. Keep. Going! Are you ready?

The Fearlessly Fertile Morning Practice

Countless studies show that the most successful people in the world have a series of things they do *before* they officially start their day. While their exact practices may vary, they start their day with intention and do things to support their awareness, focus, and well-being. Some of these people have morning practices that are as long as two hours, like tech billionaire Jack Dorsey's five-mile walk to work. Don't worry. That's not required here. I know you are busy and this may be new, so we are going to start with twenty minutes. You may shudder at the prospect of how you are going to pack another twenty minutes of activity into your life, but if you want to give yourself the chance to change the trajectory of your fertility journey, consider this the most important twenty minutes of your day. And yes, this must be done in the morning, before you do anything else. Set your alarm to go off twenty minutes earlier and get yourself to bed twenty minutes sooner.

This daily structure is intended to support you in keeping you on track for showing up strong and strategically to your journey. This is how you will begin conditioning yourself to think differently and therefore feel and behave differently, so you can achieve different results. No more wishing or hoping. There's only *do*ing. You may find that what starts out as a bit of a pain becomes your new favorite habit. It goes by quick. So here it is.

Your new morning practice consists of four steps. I strongly suggest you do them in order.

1. *Five Minutes of Visualization/Meditation*: It's undeniable based on scientific evidence that one of the most beneficial things we can do for ourselves physically and emotionally, particularly when we are under stress, is take a few minutes each day to quiet our minds. You might see the words "visualization" and "meditation" and instantly want to barf because you've tried it before and "failed." Well, the pressure is off here, love. I don't expect you to outdo His Holiness the Dalai Lama with your meditation skills. Our objective here is to give you five minutes each day to get quiet and visualize your life as you desire it. While visualization and meditation are two distinct things, I want you to allow yourself to experience both in these five minutes. Set the timer on your phone for five minutes, put on some soft music if you like, close your eyes, and get to work. Visualize your life as you desire it to be – from the family you want, to your work, home, and anything else that feels good to you. The power of visualization is something elite athletes regularly use to enhance their performance. It's muscle memory for your mind. The more often you can see it in your mind, the more likely you will be to create it in your life. Michael Phelps visualizes his races before sticking a toe in the water, and Steph Curry sees himself making thousands of three-point shots before he ever steps onto the basketball court. Then, take some time to let your mind just go quiet and be. You might drift back and forth

between the vision and quiet and that's perfectly fine. There are no hard and fast rules here, because I firmly believe that's what makes meditation so frustrating. We all worry about whether we are doing it right! Just set your timer and go.

2. ***Two Minutes of Gratitude***: Make a list of ten things you are grateful for – write them down. Just take a moment as you write each to think about the thing, person, place, experience, or what-have-you that you are grateful for. Bring the thing to mind for twelve seconds and really connect with it for that moment. Doing so really deepens the experience. This is also a chance for you to connect with and thank your Higher Power for having your back and bringing the abundance you've identified in your gratitude list into your life.

3. ***Five Minutes of Journaling***: You might not have had a journal since fourth grade, but that's okay. If this is your first time journaling, awesome! In either case, get yourself a pretty journal that makes you feel all warm and fuzzy inside. If you want to feel like a giddy little girl again, get yourself one with a lock and a unicorn on it. Don't make journaling harder than it has to be. Allow yourself to set your intention for the day in writing. In addition to writing your intention, write out anything that is on your mind as you start the day – be it feelings, a dream you had, ideas, a situation you'd like to process, and so on. Get what's on your mind out onto paper – so it can be free!

4. ***Eight Minutes of Reading***: We read all kinds of stressful things on a daily basis. This is a chance to just let your

mind relax into a book that will nourish it. Choose books that encourage you to expand your thinking, move past limiting beliefs, and keep you deeply grounded in the truth that you can create the life and journey you desire. Set your timer for eight minutes and get going.

Make the decision that you will start this morning practice tomorrow morning. Adopt a *no excuses* policy. Every minute you spend following the structure is an investment in yourself. Guard the time you carve out for this practice like a rabid pit bull.

Be an Oscar-Winning Mama

One of the biggest mistakes we make on the fertility journey is holding the feeling of being a mom hostage until our babies are in hand. Even if you've been pregnant, you tell yourself you won't get excited until the twelve-week mark, to make sure you get past the miscarriage "danger zone." The truth is, you'll just move the goalpost to your nineteen- or twenty-week anatomical scan, wanting to make sure your baby is completely healthy. Then, chances are, you'll move the goal line once again, till after thirty-two weeks, when your baby is most likely to survive in a neonatal intensive care unit if born prematurely. That's the kind of mean girl crap we pull on ourselves. We stave off the joy, excitement, and peace that is ours for the taking, because we don't want to be disappointed or have to tell others of our "failure." That's just more Saboteur nonsense that will keep you in fear, lack, and scarcity. No. More!

I want you to dust off your play-acting skills and use your powers of imagination for good. I invite you to allow yourself to think and feel as if your baby is on the way. This is more than just the "fake it till you make it" idea that you've heard before and probably blown off as delusional. Remember what you read a few pages ago about visualization and how the best athletes in the world use it to achieve their goals. By allowing yourself to act and feel as if your baby is on the way, your perspective immediately changes. Your eyes open to an entirely new set of possibilities. You can finally feel some peace and clarity. Imagine what you might see from that vantage point! Remember, we are looking to position you to be certain you are leaving no stone unturned, and that means not squandering any opportunities. Here's what that can look like in practice:

- If you haven't done so already, choose the room in your home where you plan to make the nursery.
- Clear out the closet in that room and make space for all of your baby's things.
- Allow yourself to walk down the baby aisle that you normally avoid like the plague. Give yourself permission to be in that section and familiarize yourself with the things you plan to buy this precious baby.
- Research nannies or daycare facilities close to you that you'd like to check out.
- Buy a onesie or a stuffed animal that you will give your baby. This one may make your hair stand on end, because you are "getting ahead of yourself," but that's the point. Give yourself a chance to have a tangible representation of this precious one. I can tell you that my clients who beat insane odds all do this.

I know "Acting As If" may get under your skin, because it makes you feel like a fool or perhaps as if the people around you will wonder if you've lost your marbles, but what other people think has nothing to do with you. Starving yourself of the warm, fuzzy goodness of your baby's arrival is pointless. You may tell yourself you don't want to get your hopes up, because it hurts when you are disappointed, but let's be honest, disappointment stings no matter what you do. Nothing softens the blow, so why not allow yourself to bask in the light of possibility? Remember, you already know what it feels like to let fear and doubt run the show. What do you have to lose?

Hey, Gorgeous!

I bet it's been a long time since you've seen your reflection in the mirror and felt good about what you saw. Between the way we beat ourselves up and the extra fifteen pounds we tend to carry thanks to the cocktail of fertility drugs coursing through our veins, chances are your self-image could use a bit of an upgrade. Let's set you up to repair the relationship you have with your body with two words: *Hey, gorgeous!*

The tool I am offering you here is a way to reprogram what you say to yourself when you see your reflection. By doing so, you are creating a new neuropathway in your brain associated with your own image. It's fascinating actually and insanely effective. It will feel stupid and disingenuous at first, but this is backed by science, so try it. The practice is simple. Whenever you see your reflection, whether in a mirror, on the glass as you enter a building, in your coffee, or on a passing car, I want you to say, "Hey, gorgeous!" Say it with riotous enthusiasm, even if you have to fake it. Add an accent if you wish for some sass. My personal fave is a super thick South Georgia drawl. It doesn't matter;

just say it. If you are feeling über ovaries-to-the-wall fearless, say it out loud and own it when people look at you quizzically.

This particular practice isn't about making you an impossible-to-live-with narcissistic maniac. It's about treating you and your body with the reverence you both deserve. You are made in the image of the divine. You are asking this body of yours to throw you a bone and carry the baby you long for. Why would you talk trash to her? Think about it. If you went up to one of your friends to ask them for a favor and you said, "Hey, I need you to do XYZ, but I don't respect you, trust you, or think you will be able to do it without screwing it up," how likely will they be to help you? *Right!* They will give you the finger and tell you to shove off. Why would your body do any different? She's all you've got. Treat her with respect.

Inner Power Playlist

Along the lines of what you say when you see your reflection, setting up yourself to leave no stone unturned on this journey is also about changing what you think about yourself in general. Our internal conversation is going all day. Think about what it's like to have someone's ear for each waking hour of the day. Think of the kind of influence and power you could exert. Now imagine if that access and power were used for good, instead of spewing the negativity your Saboteur loves to dish up. Exciting, right?

One of the ways that we can reprogram our beliefs about ourselves is through the repetition of affirmations. This may sound like embarrassing self-help silliness, but it's backed by science. Our brains love repetition. Instead of just saying broad things like, "I love me," the way I am going to encourage you to develop your new internal playlist is by developing five affirmations that state the specific new beliefs you desire to cultivate for yourself. In any language, the words "I am" invoke incredible meaning. Those two words together reveal the deepest beliefs we have about ourselves. Use them with wisdom and reverence. I want you to come up with "I Am" statements for each key aspect of your journey:

Relationship with Self: I am…

Relationship with Bump Squad: I am…

Relationship with Partner: I am…

Relationship with Body: I am…

Relationship with Higher Power: I am…

I know this process will challenge you. But how likely are you to be an effective advocate for yourself and your dreams if you think you are lame, unworthy, and a failure and that the Universe is working against you? Why hold on to sad sack stories about yourself? What you think and believe fuels your actions and your results. Give yourself a chance here. Write these affirmations on a small card. Put it in your pocket and say them throughout the day. Eventually you will memorize them. A great time to say them is as you are getting dressed in the morning! Between "Hey, gorgeous" and your new affirmations, your journey will turn into a high-vibe gab fest.

Is This Mine or Is This Someone Else's?

With a seemingly endless supply of turds being flung your way on this journey, there are invitations everywhere for you to slip into freak out. As you have learned thus far, your Saboteurs are all too ready to help usher you down the rabbit hole. You've got to have an arrow in your quiver that will immediately give you the perspective you need to decide if the storm headed your way is one with your name written all over it or if it's one you can rightfully dodge. The first question you want to ask is this: "Is this mine or is this someone else's?" This question is particularly critical for the lovably type A, control-freaky, get-it-done woman. Why? Being the hyper-responsible woman you are, the truth is you probably take on way more responsibility than is actually yours. Because you are so capable, you most likely jump right into a situation and go into fixer-mode, without making the perfectly legitimate inquiry of, "Is this really mine to deal with?" A ton of stress comes from the habit of taking on concerns that are not really within our purview.

One of the best examples of this is when the people in your life, whether they be the members of your Bump Squad or those on the periphery, try to smear their fear all over you. Here's what this can look like:

- Your long-faced physician, who can't seem to crack a smile, constantly reminding you that the statistics don't look good

- People saying, stupid, thoughtless, ignorant things like, "Why don't you just adopt?" (adoption is a calling, not a consolation prize)

- "Friends" telling you, "You've been through enough; isn't it time to give up?"

- People excitedly coming out of the woodwork to share fertility tales of misery and woe about their friend's cousin's uncle's hairstylist who did ten rounds of IVF, failed each time, fell into a deep depression, started smoking crack, went broke, and then was eaten alive by a pack of rabid Chihuahuas.

Too often, those around you think they are being compassionate, but they are really just smearing their fear and judgment all over you. Most people don't realize they are even doing this and would never intentionally hurt you. But there are those who think it's their job to keep your expectations "realistic," whatever that means. In either event, you've got to ask, "Is this mine?" Is your mother's belief that having five rounds of IVF is "too many" yours to manage? Does your physician's need to temper your expectations and cover their own butt have anything to do with you? Is other peoples' need for kinship through sharing their fertility misery stories yours to deal with? None of these people's concerns or motivations are really yours. Their thoughts and opinions have intrinsic value, but they are not yours to take on. You've got enough to deal with, and you have to be judicious about how you expend your energy. If something is not really yours, give it back. Don't get sucked in. Remember where you put your Velvet Rope from Chapter 5.

Acknowledge, Choose, Act

There will be times when, despite starting our days with a killer morning routine, Acting As If, acknowledging we are gorgeous, saying positive I Am statements, and noticing what's ours versus someone else's, a turd gets through. We are human. Changing what you think and believe about yourself in the context of this journey is not the same as having a lobotomy. This is why the three-step tool I'm about to teach you is so important: Acknowledge, Choose, Act. Here's how it works:

1. **Acknowledge**: When something comes up that threatens to kill your buzz on this journey, immediately acknowledge it. Denial is for the foolish and lazy. You are neither. Call it out immediately.

2. **Choose**: In full awareness of the vision you have for your journey, how do you choose to feel about the situation presented? This is where you get to exercise the most important power you have as a human being – choice. Decide how you choose to feel in that moment.

3. **Act**: Having decided how you choose to feel, take an immediate action in furtherance of that feeling. Want to feel more self-assured? Do something immediately that makes you feel more confident. Interrupt the negative pattern immediately. Get your butt up out of your chair and take action.

To clarify this even more, here's how this tool may look when applied:

1. *Acknowledge:* My annoying aunt is starting to unload another fertility horror story on me and I feel the desire to thunder-punch her in the throat.

2. *Choose:* I'm not looking to spend the rest of my childbearing years in prison, so instead of feeling rage, I choose to feel empowered.

3. *Act:* Tell your aunt that you aren't up for hearing the story. If you are in person, politely offer her a cookie, so she can flap her gums on something else. If you are on the phone, change the subject or end the call.

In this example, you can see how quickly you can change the trajectory of any given situation by exercising the power of choice and taking action. You can also see how ACA also incorporates elements of "Is This Mine or Someone Else's?" Your aunt's need to tell another fertility horror story is about her, not you. Why take that on? Stop it in its tracks and move on in three steps.

Honey Time

As we discussed in Chapter 6, the relationship you have with your partner is the foundation of the family you desire to build. You can't afford to let it be roadkill on the path to your baby. What would be the point? Instead of letting another day go by, living like roommates who have some things in common and meet up occasionally to make a baby, make a daily investment in *Honey Time*. This is about having a well-stocked store of sincere good will between the two of you when times get rough and keeping you focused on the fact that your life is now. It's a great life.

Honey Time is easy. Commit to spending fifteen minutes a day when the two of you are home just digging each other's company. Put your phones down, cut the baby talk, and put 100 percent of your attention on each other. Maybe this happens while you are making dinner, changing out of your work clothes, or settling into bed for the night. Look your partner in the eye. Reminisce about what made you two fall in love and admire what makes each other great. This doesn't have to be contrived, sappy, or filled with grand gestures. It is about getting down to the basics that keep our relationships strong and the home fires burning. Set an alarm on your phone. Do it. If you are apart, get creative!

Luxurious Self-Care

When you are watching your diet, going to endless appointments, and seemingly doing everything under the sun to get yourself ready to conceive, it can feel like you are already engaged in doing a ton of self-care. You're not. That's not really for you. It's for one of your goals, but it's really not for you. The you inside. The Luxurious Self-Care I speak of is 100 percent, unabashedly focused on you, lady. There is no end in mind other than making Mama feel amazing. One of the things I hear women across the globe say is how they feel like they've lost themselves to this journey. No more, babe. That unnecessary oversight will make you old before your time and will run you so ragged you may quietly start undermining your best efforts to get pregnant without even knowing it. Not. Good.

Luxurious Self-Care isn't necessarily about booking yourself into some swanky spa, unless of course that's your jam. Self-care is about taking care of you, whatever that may mean. Sometimes you don't even have to go anywhere. It could be giving yourself the gift of staring at the wall in silence for ten minutes when you get home, instead of immediately launching into the chaos of figuring out what's for dinner. Maybe it's super fun, easy-breezy chatter with your BFF from third grade who you can always count on. Whatever it may be, you've got to make time for it. This journey, by its very nature, is drawing on resources that you might not even know you had. You can't give to your baby, your partner, or anyone else from an empty cup. The woman who shows up to this journey in her power is well-nourished mind, body, and soul. In the space below, list ten different activities that feel like luxurious self-care to you; then decide you will make time to do at least one activity per week. My gold star overachievers will find a way to incorporate some self-care, daily!

1. _____

2. _____

3. _____

4. _____

5. _____

6. _____

7. _____

8. _____

9. _____

10. _____

My love, each of the practices and tools I have shared here is designed to help you empower your approach to this journey. Each is a way of supporting you to keep your eye on the prize and keep you focused on what really matters – taking care of you, so that you can be certain you are truly doing everything you can to bring your baby into the world with no regrets. Every moment you spend implementing, experimenting with, and allowing yourself to live what I've shared here is an investment well made. It's a chance to take the action to put yourself back into the role of leadership on this journey, where you rightfully belong. This is how you will make your decisions that set you up for success, informed. Now, get down to business.

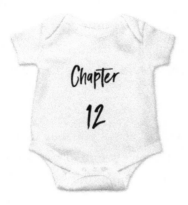

So Whatcha Gonna Do?

"In any moment of decision, the best thing you can do is the right thing, the next best thing is the wrong thing. The worst thing you can do is nothing."
— Theodore Roosevelt

At this point in our journey together, it would be no exaggeration to say that I've thrown a lot of information in your direction. There have undoubtedly been facets of your journey that perhaps you've never thought of in the way that I've presented them here. It's possible that there are even old memories that were stirred up and got you thinking, "Holy crap. That's still there?" Whatever the case may be, in addition to raising your level of awareness, I've also given you some killer tools, strategies, and ideas to work with as you move through this next phase in your journey. This brings us to a critical question: are you ready to be 100 percent certain you have done everything you can to get pregnant, harboring no regret?

Yes or No?

I know there may be part of you that's screaming "YES!" I've been doing this work long enough to also know there may be part of you leaning back in her chair thinking, "Wow, that sounds like a lot of work on top of everything else I'm doing. Can I really do this?" Who will win here, love? The part of you that knows in her soul she must give her desire to be a mom everything she's got and then some, or the one that just wants to whine, complain, and slowly give up? You might take issue with me about this binary choice, but when I look at the women I serve across the globe and to my own personal experience with success on this journey, you are either in this to win or you're not. You've got to be that hungry, that committed, and that unstoppable. You can see with what I've taught you so far; there is a path to getting there. You simply have to get out of your own way. Everything I have taught you is about taking ownership of *your* life. It's about showing the same dogged determination you've shown in all other aspects of your life and letting that fire burn for something personal and meaningful to you: being a mom. What's it going to be, my darling woman? *It's either yes or no.* The answer to this question will be found from the neck down and there's no doubt it's thundering within you as you read this. Trust it.

If at this point the answer to my question is a resounding no for you, I want to thank you for coming this far with me. It takes bravery to honor the truth within you, particularly when your truth is deciding you are not willing to go all the way for your dreams. Being 100 percent *all in* is a recipe for success, and can indeed take a lot out of you. Perhaps your reserves are depleted. I totally get it. What I would encourage you to do is revisit Chapter 4 in this book regularly. Over time, the vision you have for your journey can change. I am sure that the vision you had for yourself even one year ago is a bit different than it is today. Honor where you are and give yourself the freedom to reevaluate the situation, and perhaps change your mind. That's our prerogative as women. Just know that, if there is a day when you are ready to commit 100 percent to knowing you have done everything to get pregnant, this book, my work, and I will be here for you. It's been awesome to be part of your journey.

If you are still reading, I am going to presume your answer to my question is a resounding *yes.* This is really exciting, love. Taking this stand for yourself will have a ripple effect in your life that you can't even begin to imagine. You are about to embark on something that will represent a pivot point in your life. I know that I was scared when I made the decision that I was *all in* on my journey, which you now know means *mind and body.* This decision represents saying goodbye to victimhood and hello to the freedom that comes from taking 100 percent responsibility for your happiness and success. It means giving yourself the gift of no regret. Amen! Celebrate this.

Are You Down with DIY?

The question now becomes, how do you want to embark on this next empowered stage of your journey? Do you want to try to do it on your own, or do you want help? Let's take a look at your first option, which we will call the DIY route. When I hit rock bottom on my journey, devastated by another failed IVF cycle, I really had nowhere to turn, so I started with the DIY route. I started the slow, at times frustrating, process of beginning to educate myself. Like I had done in the early stages of my fertility journey, I began reading anything I could get my hands on, scouring the internet for answers and trying to find like-minded people on this journey who understood what I was trying to do – cultivate the thoughts and beliefs that would help support my success. God love them, but the people I surrounded myself with the most didn't know anything about personal development and looked at anything relating to it with suspicion. I didn't dare speak of what I was trying to do. Sometimes I would say I was trying to be "positive," or "improve my outlook." Most of the time I'd get a mildly patronizing, "That's nice dear," but many times I'd just get a blank stare. I decided at that point to just keep my mouth shut and keep moving forward.

Moving forward on my own was much harder than I thought. At first I figured, "I'm smart, well-educated, and persistent! I've got this." While all of those things were true, my progress was slow, frustrating, and routinely stalled. How are you supposed to solve a problem using the same thinking that created it? I didn't know what I didn't know. I'd read a book, get excited for a few days, and then find myself in a fear spiral all over again. I'd read an inspirational quote online in some group, want to have it tattooed to my body, and then find myself wanting to jump out the ground-floor window of my office because I heard that another annoying, "undeserving" woman in my office was pregnant

– effortlessly, of course. Was that woman annoying and undeserving? Absolutely not! She deserved her happiness, but without accountability and someone helping me remove the blocks that were getting in my way, I kept falling back into the mean, destructive patterns I couldn't seem to shake. That's the inherent trouble with DIY. The utter lack of accountability, slow progress, and lack of outside mentorship – particularly from someone who has lived this journey – is a formula for monumental failure. The nature of limiting beliefs and how deeply ingrained they may be make them extremely difficult to root out on our own. Your Saboteurs have been your old friends for decades. They will resist the eviction notice you try to give them. Indeed, we can become aware of them, but beating them at their own game, without help, can make this process seem insurmountable. Remember that part of you that was tempted to say, "Wow. That sounds like a lot of work?" This is where it can take hold and sabotage your DIY efforts with the blink of an eye. This is where you'll catch yourself saying counterproductive things like, "I have so many other things to do on top of this" and then finding yourself slowly drifting away from the truths I shared in this book until you find yourself right back in the pit of despair. DIY is a great place to start, but your Saboteurs love it because it can mean job security for them. Worst of all, the DIY approach perpetuates the notion that you "have" to do this on your own. Certainly there is something satisfying about doing things on our own, but when it comes to achieving the biggest, most meaningful goals, why make things harder and slower than they have to be? That question leads us to another reality every woman faces when she takes a stand for having no regrets on her journey.

B.S. Can Still Get in Your Way

Even if you follow the steps I've shared in this book, there will be obstacles at every turn. When we take big leaps, it can feel like God and the Universe are testing us at every turn, asking, "How bad do you want this?" If you are committed to success on this journey, your answer must be unequivocally, "Bad!" That means you must be ready to face resistance. I love you and want to keep it real, so I will break it down for you here, how these obstacles may look. A winning strategy on this journey requires that you must rise to the occasion when they appear.

Let's start with the very first step I shared in Chapter 4: The Reset. This is where you learned how to gain a new, more strategic perspective on the complete set of facts that form the body of your journey. Taking this wider, more intellectually honest perspective can mind-blowing, because it can feel like you are seeing an aspect of your journey you didn't really know existed. That being said, this leveled-up awareness can be like the new girl in town. She is pretty, wildly interesting, and seemingly exotic, but no one feels like they can trust her yet. Trust takes time and consistent reinforcement – particularly when the "new girl" is shaking things up in your world. Like a plane, which expends most of its fuel at take-off, at this stage you will find yourself doing some major heavy lifting to maintain this wiser perspective. Even though you know what I am teaching is smart, effective, and proven, the temptation will be to scrap the take-off because it's new and hard, at least in the beginning. This is why having a coach, who has mastered this work and has been like air traffic control guiding women through this step and on to fertility success, is so critical.

The next obstacle comes in Chapter 5, when I teach you how to form, manage, and lead the Bump Squad that can carry you to victory. Plain and simple, the obstacle here is that, with decades of conditioning that tells you people in white lab coats have the final say, it's way too easy to chicken out. Becoming the leader of your team and having to assert yourself in an area of your life where you feel more like the water girl than the star quarterback can make you feel adrift and foolish. Having an expert Bump Squad curator by your side who has successfully guided women to creating winning teams with a Western, alternative, or combined approach is like money in the bank. It's particularly awesome when that same coach is the expert physicians across the globe turn to when developing their own bullet-proof fertility mindset. As you know from your study of this step, your Bump Squad includes friends, family, and coworkers – and establishing new boundaries with them during this chapter in your life. The most challenging obstacle in that realm is effectively communicating and consistently enforcing, as well as navigating the nuances of those boundaries with people who may bristle boisterously against them. Support, guidance, and the level-headed vision of an unrelated third party with this exact experience is vital.

When becoming the woman you truly desire to be in your partnership, as we discussed in Chapter 6, the critical challenge is having the discipline to view your most intimate relationship in an objective way. It's a daunting task that is rarely accomplished without support – because of how hard it is to view an incredibly emotional subject without being caught up in the emotion – especially when the subject is *your partnership!* Even as a former prosecutor, highly skilled in the art of the poker face, with thousands of hours of coaching under my belt, I too need the support of my coach to find objectivity when working toward goals in my own relationship. This becomes an even more important consideration when the relationship is already strained due to neglect, lack of communication, or both of you feeling so paralyzed you can't make a move in any direction. In matters of the heart, level heads prevail. If you are committed to liberating your relationship from Cell Mate Creep, have an "escapee" show you the way.

Creating a new vision for living your fertility journey, which includes changing what you think and believe about yourself like you did in Chapter 7, can feel like idiotic, delusional, wishful thinking when by most commonly accepted measures you are *really bad* at making babies. The obstacle you face in this step is building the muscle it takes to lead with that vision, *before* it's your reality. It requires that you take control of what you think and believe, which is the exact opposite of what most people do in their lives. The idea that you have the qualities of the people you most admire or that you have fearlessness within you may run in stark contrast with the experiences you've had on this journey. There will be temptation everywhere to look at the vision you've created and tell yourself that you just don't have what it takes. Without strong, consistent accountability, you are less likely to finish what you start here. Think about how different your workout is when you have an instructor than when you try to do an exercise video at home! Make no mistake: for your mind, changing your self image in the context of this journey *will be a work out*. This is why those who are truly committed to success hire coaches. Any world-class athlete will tell you their success depends as much as their ability to "see" themselves winning as it does physically executing that win on the field. Can you imagine Venus or Serena showing up to Wimbledon without their coaches?

In Chapter 8, when we take on the subject of your Saboteurs, the obstacle will be the ability to effectively spot them in the first place. Now you might take issue with this by pointing to the fact that you actually listed your Top Three. That's an awesome starting point, but the real work is facing the megalodon of a Saboteur that's lurking behind the scenes. Your darkest Saboteurs have Machiavellian cunning. They are smart enough to toss you low-hanging fruit like failure, age, and being "good enough." I call these low-hanging fruit because they are "safe," accessible, and relatively easy to discuss for the work in this book. It's the Saboteurs *you didn't know to write down* that are waiting in the wings to betray you. More often than not, our most dangerous Saboteurs can be virtually invisible to us. We normalize their existence and perhaps even see them as stories that serve us, because they keep us "honest," "on our toes," and high-achieving. Powerful, probing questions from an expert mentor adept at sniffing out your most hardcore Saboteurs can help you end the cycle of sabotage for good. When it comes to your Saboteurs, go big or go home.

With embracing the fearlessness that you discovered in Chapter 9, the challenge will be your willingness to trust this inner wisdom enough to stand alone. Taking this step means you are no longer looking outside of yourself for answers. Your choices are informed by the only authority that really matters:

you. This can be an incredibly lonely place, as it means letting go of the past, aligning with your values, possibly being unpopular, and daring to live this journey by heart. It takes incredible courage to stand by your internally guided decisions. Trusting yourself to this degree and releasing your familiar grip on the conventional wisdom of seeking answers from others can feel like free fall. Smart women have a mentor by their side to help them spot the net when it appears.

The faith I encourage you to explore, build, and lovingly cultivate in Chapter 10 will be challenged at every turn, by something you love with all of your heart: control. Faith by its very nature requires you to relinquish it, or at least your sense of it. We love the comfort of lulling ourselves into believing we have control of the world around us, when in fact the only real control you have is over yourself. Even if your faith is in good shape, admit it: there's part of you that operates like God and the Universe need your help to nudge them along. It's a hard habit to break, particularly when you are road-weary and afraid. A compassionate mentor who has done the work to rebuild her own faith when it felt almost impossible to do so can help soften your gaze so you can see the blessings all around.

While I have given you some incredible tools in Chapter 11, without the support to apply them to your unique situation, will you actually use them to their best advantage? Unlikely. In clutch moments, you might remember a few ideas, you may even start your daily practice, but until you get each and every practice into your bones, which requires the kind of consistency fostered by accountability, these tools will simply remain in the confines of these pages, instead of being fully incorporated into your life.

The Truth About Women Who Succeed on This Journey

You will have many forces working against you, love. You will likely want to quit. You will question the wisdom of this undertaking. You might even question me, but here's a reality that you must face: Women who succeed on this journey have the mindset for it. They are holding babies today because they didn't punk out. They brought everything they had to this journey, mind and body. They refused to rest on the laurels of expecting medicine to come save them and they did not wait for anyone's permission to live their dream. They made a decision to take extreme responsibility and have no regrets. When you decide that you will no longer let fear, negativity, doubt, or excuses get in your way, you will see opportunities you had no idea were right under your nose. You will get intuitive hits that will lead you confidently in the direction that feels right to you, instead of feeling confined by skewed statistics, fear-mongering, and lack-based thinking that has failed to put a baby in your arms. Taking control of what you think and believe on this journey will give you a chance to live it on your terms – dare I say confidently. By doing this work, you give yourself the chance to be the woman who may not know when or exactly how, but *knows* her baby is coming. Taking control of what you think and believe can give you a delightfully unfair advantage. You can be the happiest mama-to-be you know.

The Risk of Doing Nothing

While it's true, you can live your journey without having your mindset on board, the risk you run is the crushing pain of regret that comes from leaving a gaping hole in your strategy. With over eighty medical schools in the United States alone teaching the power of the mind-body connection, why not have this strategy tucked in your back pocket? You know your mindset is not where you want it to be. You wouldn't be reading this book if it was. There's part of you that is deeply afraid of looking back on this journey and knowing you were your own worst enemy. This breaks my heart, because while we can't always control the circumstances around us, we can control how we show up. We are the common denominator in our lives. We have the power to control what we think and believe. Why let something that is so clearly within our control sabotage the thing we want most in this life? I've said it before, and it bears repeating now: there is nothing more expensive than regret.

Decide now that you will apply my Fearlessly Fertile™ Methodology and get the expert support that can help you clear a path to your baby, leaving no stone unturned. If you are ready, I'm here.

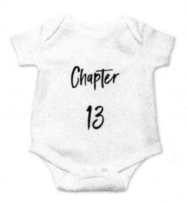

Chapter

13

Time to Fly, Mama

"The greatest glory in living lies not in never falling,
but in rising every time we fall."
— Ralph Waldo Emerson

Every woman's fertility journey is a gift. It is a chance to dig deeper, clear out the cobwebs, and forge a path through the unknown, to become the woman she desires to be: mother, partner, daughter, sister, friend, coworker, manifester of miracles. I know that may sound a little like a Pollyanna platitude, but by now you should know that's not how I roll. It's simply the truth, if you are willing to see it. It's a reclamation in many ways, not only of who you are, but what you believe.

Each step I have shared with you in our journey together is about developing a deeper relationship with truth – the complete truth, not just what is thrust into your face by those around you. It's the truth you dare to hold on to when everyone around you is telling you that you are a fool and should just give up. We both know that's not truth. You've made it this far, love; don't you dare do that.

You are a woman with a dream who is facing what will likely be one of the most challenging chapters of her life. Mad respect to you, Mama, for stepping up to it. I hope you know now, you are definitely not alone. Let me remind you that you have a history of success – just look at the life you live now. It's a testament to that fact. Even if you feel like a loser right now, you've got to know that's not the whole picture. This journey is part of your life, it's not the sum total of it.

The ideas, wisdom, tools, and practices I have shared in this book will help you reconnect with that. While we are indeed different people, we have a shared experience. In sharing mine with you, it is my sincere hope that you can see that even the most stubborn, type A, lovably control-freaky of us can triumph on this journey, in the face of insane odds. Whether you've boiled black chickens or not, I feel you, girl. What I lived through is the "why" behind what I do. I swore that if I figured out the missing piece to setting myself up for success on this journey, I'd shout it from the rooftops and share it with anyone who would listen. This book is one of the ways I am making good on that promise, in addition to building my coaching practice, online courses, group programs, retreats, and podcast that is serving women on this journey all over the world. This work is about becoming your own insurance policy for fertility success.

Your job now, Mama, is to bring all of the pieces of this process together. Be honest about your wins and the lessons that have shown up along the way. This is what any smart warrior would do.

Assemble your crew of supporters who will have your back, come what may. Commit to making your connection with your partner a priority. Embrace your vision, not worst-case scenarios. Take control of the one thing in this life you can control: you. By applying what I've shared in this book you have a chance to completely reshape the road forward so that lame, fear-based, short-sighted decision-making can stop blocking you from your baby. Say goodbye to the tired, broken-down victim story that will mercilessly hold your dreams hostage to other people's opinions, statistics, and the cowardice of naysayers.

Remember that at any given moment, you have the power to choose your vision over your fear. You can recover from any fall. You can get back on track. See how unstoppable you can be? It's about progress, not perfection, baby.

Don't forget that faith lights your baby's path home. Open your heart to seeing the signs everywhere. My darling, you are and will be, well taken care of.

The tools I have given you as a starting point must be applied with open-minded consistency. Let them be fun. Celebrate and delight in each millimeter of progress you make. Remember, this is about bringing your very best self to this journey, so you can cover your bases, mind and body, to support your success. It's the simple and effective recipe for the sweet confidence you daydream about. Claim it, sister. It's yours for the taking. It's your birthright.

Love, my wish for you is that you can see that you are the foundation for your success on this journey. What you think and believe can be more powerful than any pill someone wants you to pop or hormone someone wants you to inject. *You are your own fertility miracle drug.* Learning to think about yourself and your fertility journey in a new way, isn't about never having failures again, or never spending another moment afraid. Don't set yourself up with that ridiculous expectation. What you've learned here is about personal mastery. It's about living this journey on your terms, and being the woman with the guts to shape her own fertility destiny, no BS, no excuses, and absolutely no regret. Go live your dreams, Mama.

Acknowledgments

To say my fertility journey was a pivotal moment in my life would be a ridiculous understatement. In no uncertain terms, it burned every belief I had about the way the world is *supposed to* work to cinders. As painful as this chapter in my life was, I thank God and the Universe for the gift of it. My journey was the chance to rebuild my life – based upon truth, intuition, faith, gratitude, freedom, responsibility, and the unwavering belief that even with all of my imperfections, I am worthy of the dreams that stir in my heart.

This transformation would not have been possible without the love and support of those who could see what I couldn't. To all of you, I am eternally grateful.

To Brandon and Asher, while this book is dedicated to you, I must acknowledge the countless sacrifices you've made in support of "Mama's Work." Thank you for your patience while I am on the phone, making dinner while I work into the wee hours of the night, holding down the fort while I travel, putting up with my moments of crazy, and always being ready to drop everything to be my most trusted counsel. I love you both beyond words.

To Mom, Dad, Mike, Anna, Patti, and David. I am honored to call you my family. Thank you for all of the loving encouragement and unwavering support. To my family on the gorgeous island of Guam, Si Yu'us Ma'ase.

To Diego, Tiberius, Shreddy, Jake, Keeno, Shelby, Vincent, and Big Red. There's no question who rescued who.

To my alpha-female ride or die sisters from another mother, Karina, Heather, Kim, Tracy, Sue, Victoria, and Rachel, thank you for always having wine, words of wisdom, bail money, and a getaway car at the ready. Counting you as my dearest friends is one of the great joys of my life.

To my mentors and teachers, Gina, Sonni, Susan, and Angela, thank you for being the wise, kind, passionate, take no BS trailblazers you are. You paved and lit the way for me. Your courage, ingenuity, counsel, and unique ability to yank genius out of me is nothing short of amazing. Thank you for helping me manifest my dreams.

To those whose work inspired me when I needed it most, Bernie Siegel, MD, Wayne Dyer, Bob Proctor, Tony Robbins, Pastor Joel Osteen, Marianne Williamson, Jen Sincero, Napoleon Hill, Wallace Wattles, Emmett Fox, Joyce Meyer, and Neville Goddard.

To Joanne, thank you for the love and support of my work from the very start. You believed in me back when I couldn't quite articulate exactly what I did. Your kindness, patience, and generosity set all of this in motion. If someone checked you for angel's wings, there is no question they would find them. Mad love and respect.

To my editor Bethany, thank you for supporting my vision and caring enough to ruthlessly demand more from me. It has been and honor and pleasure.

Thank you to The Author Incubator team, as well as to David Hancock and the Morgan James Publishing team for helping me bring this book to print.

To Wendy, the images you have captured of me and my family are the stuff of dreams. Your artistry has helped me create a brand I love. Thank you for always reminding to wiggle my toes and take a deep breath. I can't wait to see what we create next.

To Andy, your compassionately firm nutrition coaching not only guided me through my incredibly healthy miracle preg-nancy, but helped me stay properly energized through the writing of this book. At its core, your work is about helping women make their dreams come true. Thank you for making food fun again.

To my ladies all over the world, my love for you is why I do what I do. You are an endless source of inspiration. Being part of your fertility journey and having the honor of being by your side as you make your Mama dreams come true *is my dream come true.*

To each of my Unicorns who bestowed upon me the honor of sharing your remarkable stories in this book, I love you to the moon and back. Your kindness and generosity will inspire other women to keep saying their YES. Thank you for helping me bring this book to life.

To the doubters, naysayers, and fear-mongerers I met along the way, thank you for awakening the Kraken of defiance within me. It helped bring me into alliance with my wisest, most confident self, and as a result, I am living a life beyond my wildest dreams.

Thank You!

Wondering what to do now that you've read the book? Don't worry, love, I've got your back.

Get my **FREE Fearlessly Fertile Method™ Kick Start Audio Course** as bonus for reading this book and inviting me into your journey.

In this laser focused thirty-minute course, I will teach you powerful next steps that will help you gain unshakable confidence that you have *all* of your bases covered – mind and body – so you can start living your fertility journey with *no regret*.

My clients all over the world have used what I teach to help them beat incredible odds. You can too!

In this bonus course, you will get these insider secrets:

- Learn what a woman who beats the odds is "really thinking" as she moves through each of the steps in my Fearlessly Fertile Method™,
- The single most important decision you must make if you are truly committed to fertility success, *and*
- The big YES my clients and I all said that helped us make the seemingly "impossible," possible on our journeys!

You will also receive a helpful worksheet to accompany your Kick Start Audio Course.

To get your Bonus Audio Course and Worksheet go to: https://www.frommaybetobaby.com/bookgift

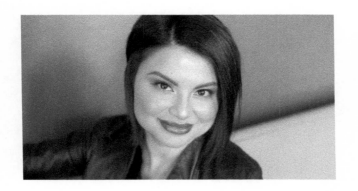

About the Author

Rosanne Austin, author of *Am I The Reason I'm Not Getting Pregnant*, is a former state prosecutor turned Fertility Fairy Godmother. She has helped women around the world get pregnant in the face of overwhelming odds. Rosanne walks the talk, having given birth to her miracle son at age forty-three, despite years of fertility treatment failure. With her book, podcast, online courses, and retreats, Rosanne helps her clients become the moms they were meant to be. She resides with her family in Eagle, Idaho.

Lightning Source UK Ltd.
Milton Keynes UK
UKHW012208040820
367662UK00010B/99